Guide to the preparation, use and quality assurance of blood components

Recommendation No. R (95) 15

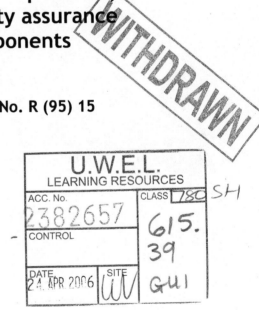

12th edition

Council of Europe Publishing

French edition:

Guide pour la préparation, l'utilisation et l'assurance de qualité des composants sanguins

ISBN-10: 92-871-5883-5
ISBN-13: 978-92-871-5883-3

Cover painting: water colour - Eloïse Cuny, aged five
Cover design: Graphic Design Workshop, Council of Europe

Council of Europe Publishing
F-67075 Strasbourg Cedex
http://book.coe.int

ISBN-10: 92-871-5884-3
ISBN-13: 978-92-871-5884-0
© Council of Europe, January 2006
Printed at the Council of Europe

Foreword

Founded in 1949, the Council of Europe is the oldest and largest of all European institutions and now numbers 46 member states*. One of its founding principles is that of increasing co-operation between member states to improve the quality of life for all Europeans.

Within this context of intergovernmental co-operation in the field of health, the Council of Europe has consistently selected ethical problems for study. The most important such ethical issue relates to the non-commercialisation of human substances i.e. blood, organs and tissues.

With regard to blood transfusion, co-operation among member states started back in the 1950s. From the outset, the activities were inspired by the following guiding principles: promotion of voluntary, non-remunerated blood donation, mutual assistance, optimal use of blood and blood products and protection of the donor and the recipient.

The first result of this co-operation was the adoption of the European Agreement on the Exchange of Therapeutic Substances of Human Origin (European Treaty Series, No. 26) in 1958. It was followed by the European Agreement on the exchange of blood grouping reagents (European Treaty Series, No. 39) and of tissue-typing reagents (European Treaty Series, No. 84) in 1962 and 1976 respectively.

Around these three Agreements, the Council of Europe has established a blood transfusion programme whose aim is to ensure good quality of blood and blood products.

Since then, the Council of Europe has adopted a number of recommendations covering ethical, social, scientific and training aspects of blood transfusion. Whereas Agreements are binding on the States that ratify them, recommendations are policy statements to governments proposing a common course of action to be followed. Major recommendations include Recommendation No. R (88) 4 on the responsibilities of Health Authorities in the field of blood transfusion or this Recommendation No. R (95) 15, which contains as technical appendix guidelines on the use, preparation and quality assurance of blood components.

---

*　　*Albania, Andorra, Armenia, Austria, Azerbaijan, Belgium, Bosnia and Herzegovina, Bulgaria, Croatia, Cyprus, Czech Republic, Denmark, Estonia, Finland, France, Georgia, Germany, Greece, Hungary, Iceland, Ireland, Italy, Latvia, Liechtenstein, Lithuania, Luxembourg, Malta, Moldova, Monaco, Netherlands, Norway, Poland, Portugal, Romania, Russia, San Marino, Serbia and Montenegro, Slovakia, Slovenia, Spain, Sweden, Switzerland, "the former Yugoslav Republic of Macedonia", Turkey, Ukraine, United Kingdom*

Work on Recommendation No. R (95) 15 started in 1986, when the Select Committee of Experts on Quality Assurance in Blood Transfusion Services published proposals on quality assurance in blood transfusion services. Based on these proposals, the Select Committee produced a more comprehensive guide on blood components in 1995. The immediate success and acceptability of this document was such that the Committee of Ministers adopted it as a technical appendix to what then became Recommendation No. R (95) 15.

Recommendation No. R (95) 15 also states that its technical appendix will be regularly up-dated to keep it in line with scientific progress. The Committee is now charged with producing annual up-dates. This is the 12th edition of Recommendation No. R (95) 15. Major changes are outlined below. Further amendments take into account comments made during the consultation procedure of the 11th edition where National Health Authorities as well as interested parties were invited to comment on the proposed text. During the elaboration of the 4th edition this consultation procedure was introduced for the first time with great success. It is on the basis of this procedure that the publication of future editions is envisaged.

The members of the Committee of Experts on Quality Assurance in Blood Transfusion Services who worked on this 12th edition of Recommendation No. R (95) 15 are listed in the acknowledgements.

Major changes introduced in this 12th Edition

PART B - Blood collection - Chapter 1 on *Selection of Donors*

In Part B, *Considerations specific for donors of different types of components* a paragraph on iron deficiency has been added;

The section on malaria under the heading *Infectious diseases* has been completely modified.

PART D - Technical procedures

Chapter 23 - *Screening for infectious markers*

Paragraph 6 on *Quality control of malarial antibody testing* has been updated.

Chapter 24 on *Control of equipment* has been partly modified.

Chapter 27 on *Statistical process control* has been completely modified.

PART E - Transfusion practices

Chapter 30 on *Haemovigilance* has been completely modified.

APPENDIX 1 (list of definitions)

The definitions of *adverse event*, *adverse reaction* and *blood bag* have been added.

CONTENTS

Page

COUNCIL OF EUROPE

COMMITTEE OF MINISTERS

RECOMMENDATION No. R (95) 15

OF THE COMMITTEE OF MINISTERS
TO MEMBER STATES

ON THE PREPARATION, USE AND
QUALITY ASSURANCE
OF BLOOD COMPONENTS

*(Adopted by the Committee of Ministers on 12 October 1995
at the 545th meeting of the Ministers' Deputies)*

The Committee of Ministers, under the terms of Article 15.*b* of the Statute of the Council of Europe;

Considering that the aim of the Council of Europe is to achieve greater unity between its members and that this aim may be pursued, *inter alia*, by the adoption of common action in the health field;

Recalling its Resolution (78) 29 on harmonisation of legislations of member states relating to removal, grafting and transplantation human substances;

Recalling also its Recommendations No. R (80) 5 concerning blood products for the treatment of haemophiliacs, No. R (81) 14 on preventing the transmission of infectious diseases in the international transfer of blood, its components and derivatives, No. R (84) 6 on the prevention of the transmission of malaria by blood transfusion, No. R (85) 12 on the screening of blood donors for the presence of Aids markers, No. (86) 6 on guidelines for the preparation, quality control and use of fresh frozen plasma, No. R (88) 4 on the responsibilities of health authorities in the field of blood transfusion and No. R (93) 4 concerning clinical trials involving the use of components and fractionated products derived from human blood or plasma;

Taking into account the Council Directive 89/38/EEC extending the scope of Directives 65/65/EEC and 75/319/EEC on the approximation of provisions laid down by law, regulation or administrative action relating to proprietary medical products and laying down special provisions for medicinal products derived from human blood or human plasma;

Taking into account Agreement No. 26 on the exchange of therapeutic substances of human origin;

Considering the importance of blood components in modern haemotherapy and the necessity to ensure their safety, efficacy and quality;

Considering that such components are of human origin and that hence specific ethical and technical principles have to be taken into account;

Considering that biotechnology does not provide substitutes for most blood products;

Convinced, therefore, of the need to provide health authorities, transfusion services as well as hospital blood banks and clinical users with a set of guidelines for the preparation, use and the quality assurance of blood components;

Aware that the *Guide to the preparation, use and quality assurance of blood components* published by the Council of Europe has already become the generally-accepted European standard and that it is therefore appropriate to give a legal basis to this guide;

Considering that this guide will be regularly updated by the committee of experts of the Council of Europe;

Recommends that the governments of member states take all necessary measures and steps to ensure that the preparation, use and quality control of blood components are carried out in accordance with the guidelines set out in the appendix to this recommendation.

APPENDIX

to Recommendation No. R (95) 15 on the preparation, use and quality assurance of blood components

APPENDIX

to Recommendation No. R (95) 15 on the preparation, use and quality assurance of blood components

Introduction

The purpose of this recommendation is to provide transfusion services with a set of guidelines and principles relating to the preparation, use and quality assurance of blood components. These guidelines should form the basis for standard operating procedures (SOPs).

These guidelines and descriptions of the different blood components should also be of value to hospital blood banks and the clinical users of these therapeutic products. As these guidelines were originally and primarily designed to provide information on quality assurance, some emphasis is to be expected on this aspect including the selection of donors, the control of laboratory reagents and competency testing of staff carrying out the procedures necessary for the safe preparation, selection and transfusion of blood and its components.

This recommendation covers all of the normal components of blood which will be prepared at a routine blood transfusion service. It does not cover plasma products obtained by fractionation. In respect of plasma-derived products, technical matters are addressed by the European Pharmacopoeia. The European Union has a substantial body of legislation regarding pharmaceutical products including plasma-derived products.

On 27 January 2003, the European Union adopted Directive 2002/98/EC on setting standards of quality and safety for the collection, testing, processing, storage and distribution of human blood and blood components. As regards technical requirements to be set under Article 29 of the said Directive, the European Commission and the Council of Europe work closely together to ensure that these requirements are compatible with the ones described in the Guide.

Whereas blood establishments in EU Member States are required to comply with legislation derived from the European Commission Directives, this Guide is intended to facilitate ongoing improvements on the preparation, use and quality assurance of blood components through education and the provision of non-binding recommendations and may differ in some respects from those contained in the European Commission Directives.

The Council of Europe wishes to express its gratitude to the European Commission who contributed a substantial amount of information to revise the Chapter 30 on *Haemovigilance*, by giving its approval to use information from the "Feasibility project on the establishment of a Haemovigilance Network in the European Community"*.

This Guide provides information and additional guidance on best practices consistent with current scientific understanding and expert opinion. At any given time, implementation of these recommendations may vary among Member States and individual blood establishments, and alternative procedures, practices and standards may be in place.

It is inevitable, even in the best of laboratories, that some materials will fail some of the tests, and a strict protocol should be drawn up showing action to be taken in such an eventuality. It is essential that all staff in a blood transfusion service be trained to accept quality control as a welcome and necessary part of everyday work. It is useful to cultivate a positive attitude towards the detection and correction of errors though the emphasis is on the prevention of problems and the production of blood components. A sensible scheme of rotation of junior staff between routine departments and the quality control department may help to foster such an attitude.

In July 2004 the Council of Europe published the second edition of a new Guide on safety and quality assurance for organs, tissues and cells. Following its publication, any reference to haematopoietic progenitor cells was deleted in this Guide on the preparation, use and quality assurance of blood components.

---

* Carried out by the HAEMAN Consortium for the European Commission under Contract SOC 96 201709 05F01(96PRVF1-036-0).

PART A:
Quality System
for blood establishments

Quality System for blood establishments

1.   Introduction

This chapter explains the contents and background of the proposal for the Quality System for Blood Establishments, including the activities to be included in this system and the subjects to be addressed in the quality system.

The proposed Quality System is based on the principles of good practice and quality management, as described in the EU GMP guidelines and ISO 9000-series standards.

2.   The Quality System

In the quality system for blood establishments the following processes of blood establishments must be described*:

1.   Quality management and process control;

2.   Personnel and organisation;

3.   Premises, including mobile sites;

4.   Equipment and materials;

5.   Documentation;

6.   Donor session;

7.   Processing;

8.   Storage and distribution;

9.   Quality monitoring;

10.   Quality control;

11.   Contract management;

12.   Deviations, complaints, adverse events or reactions, recall, corrective and preventive actions;

13.   Self-inspection, audits and improvement.

---

*   These are minimum requirements. It is possible to add other items, such as waste management, (inter-) national guidelines.

The quality system is dedicated to the quality and safety of blood and blood components and to customer satisfaction. The system includes an evaluation and continuous improvement mechanism.

2.1   Quality management change control and validation

General

Quality is the responsibility of all persons involved in the processes of the blood establishments. Management is responsible for a systematic approach towards quality and the implementation and maintenance of a quality management system.

The quality system should involve all activities that determine the quality policy, objectives and responsibilities, and implement them by means of quality planning, quality control, quality assurance and quality improvement in order to ensure the quality and safety of blood and blood components and to fulfil customer satisfaction.

Within any blood establishment there should be an independent function with the responsibility of fulfilling Quality Assurance and Quality Control responsibilities*. The Quality Assurance function should be involved in all quality-related matters and review and approve all appropriate quality related documents.

Quality assurance

The quality assurance system should ensure that all critical processes are specified in appropriate instructions and are performed in accordance with the principles of Good Practice and comply with the appropriate regulations. Management should review the system at regular intervals to verify the effectiveness of the system and introduce corrective measures if deemed necessary.

Change control

A formal change control system should be in place to plan, evaluate and document all changes that may affect the quality, traceability, availability or effect of components or safety of components, donors or patients. The potential impact of the proposed change should be evaluated. The need for additional testing and validation should be determined.

Every blood establishment should have a general policy regarding validation of equipment, facilities, processes, automated systems and laboratory tests. The formal objective of validation is to ensure compliance with the intended use and regulatory requirements. Validation is more than simply testing a

---

*   Fulfilling the responsibility does not necessarily mean that the activities should be performed also by that function. It means a responsibility for the processes to be performed.

process, system or laboratory test. In addition, validation may demonstrate control, generate knowledge and establish future requirements on e.g. calibration and maintenance of equipment, internal quality control and training of personnel. The objective of validation is to produce documented evidence that provides high level of assurance that all parts related to the use of a process or system will work correctly and consistently. Validation should be performed on all new processes and systems that are considered critical with special emphasis on automated processes and systems. Furthermore, all existing processes and systems should be constantly monitored and periodically evaluated to maintain their validated status.

2.2   Personnel and organisation

General

Personnel should be available in sufficient number and be qualified to perform their tasks. They should have appropriate qualifications and experiences and should be provided with initial and continued training in order to assure the quality and safety of blood and blood components.

Only persons that are authorised by defined procedures and documented as such should be involved in the collection, manufacturing and distribution processes, including quality control and quality assurance.

Tasks and responsibilities

The tasks and responsibilities should be clearly documented and understood. All personnel should have clear, documented and up to date job descriptions. There should be an organisation chart showing the hierarchical structure of the blood establishment and clear delineation of lines of responsibilities.

Key personnel include:

- a Responsible Person;
- a Processing or Operations Manager;
- a Quality Assurance Manager.

The Responsible Person should have appropriate qualifications.

The Quality Assurance Manager and Processing or Operations Manager should be different individuals, functioning independently.

The Quality Assurance Manager is responsible for ensuring that there are appropriate systems and protocols in place for the safe and secure release of all materials, equipment, reagents and blood and blood components.

Delegation of responsibilities should only be given to individuals who have been trained for the task. Delegation should be in written form and be reviewed on a regular basis.

Training and competency evaluation

All personnel should receive initial and continued training appropriate to their specific tasks, which cover the relevant principles and practices of transfusion medicine. All personnel should have a competency evaluation appropriate to their specific tasks and should at least include:

- good practice;
- relevant knowledge in microbiology and hygiene.

Training and competency should be documented and training records should be maintained. The contents of training programs must be periodically reviewed and the effectiveness of training courses should be periodically assessed.

2.3   Premises, including mobile sites

General

Premises should be located, constructed, adapted and maintained to suit the operations to be carried out. Premises should be designed to permit effective cleaning and maintenance to minimise risk of contamination. The workflow in an area should be arranged in a logical sequence to minimise the risk of errors. Working areas should not be used as passageway.

The area for blood donors should be separated from all processing areas. The area for donor selection should allow confidential personal interviews with due regard for donor and personnel safety.

The premises used for the processing of blood components meant for transfusion in an open process should be in accordance with Good Manufacturing Practice.

A less stringent environment may be acceptable if in combination with additional safety measures, such as preparing the blood component within a specific time before transfusion or immediately after processing applying storage conditions that are unfavourable to microbial growth. Personnel performing open processing should wear appropriate clothing and should receive regular training in aseptic manipulations. Aseptic processing should be validated.

Laboratory areas should be separated from the processing areas.

Ancillary areas should be separated from other areas.

Washing and toilet facilities and, if required, facilities for changing should be adequate.

Processing and storage areas

Storage conditions should be controlled, monitored and checked. Appropriate alarms should be present and regularly checked; the checks should be recorded. Appropriate actions on alarms should be defined.

Intermediate storage and transport should be carried out under defined conditions to ensure that set requirements are met.

Each area of processing and storage should be secured against the entry of unauthorised persons and should be used only for the intended purpose.

Storage areas should provide effective segregation of quarantined and released materials or components. There should be a separate area for rejected components and material.

Mobile sites

Before premises are accepted for mobile donor sessions their suitability must be assessed against the following criteria:

- the size to allow proper operation and ensure donor privacy;

- safety for staff and donors;

- the presence of ventilation, electrical supply, lighting, hand washing facilities, reliable communication, blood storage and transport.

2.4   Equipment and materials

All equipment should be designed, validated and maintained to suit its intended purpose and should not present any unacceptable risks to donors or operators.

Maintenance, cleaning and calibration should be performed regularly and recorded.
Instructions for use, maintenance, service, cleaning and sanitation should be available according to the instructions for use and operator's manual.
There should be procedures for each type of equipment, detailing the action to be taken when malfunctions or failures occur.

New and repaired equipment should meet qualification requirements when installed and authorised before use. Qualification results should be documented.

Only reagents and materials from approved suppliers that meet the documented requirements and specifications should be used.

The contracting process should include:

- Checks prior to awarding the contract to help ensure suppliers meet the organisation needs;
- Appropriate checks on received goods to confirm they meet specifications;
- The requirement for manufacturers to provide a certificate of analysis for critical material
- Checks to ensure that in use goods continue to meet specification;
- Regular contact with suppliers to help understand and resolve problems.

Inventory records should be kept for traceability. Critical materials should be released under the responsibility of QA function before use. The actual release may be performed by an authorised person under the guidance of a validated information technology system.

2.5 Documentation

General

Each activity which may affect the quality of the blood and blood components should be documented and recorded as a Standard Operating Procedure (SOP). This documentation should include an SOP governing development and revision of SOPs. This documentation will ensure that work performed is standardised and that there is traceability of all steps in the process. Procedures should be designed, developed, validated and personnel trained in a consistent manner.

A document control system should be established for review, revision history and archival of documents including SOPs. It should include a distribution list. The documentation should allow all steps and all data to be checked. All documentation should be traceable and reliable. All changes to documents should be acted upon promptly and should be reviewed, dated and signed by an authorised person.

Computerised systems

All software, hardware and backup procedures should be validated before use and checked at least once a year to ensure reliability. Hardware and software should be protected against unauthorised use or changes.

There should be procedures for each type of soft- and hardware, detailing the action to be taken when malfunctions or failures occur. A backup procedure should be in place to prevent loss of records at expected and unexpected down time or function failures.

Changes in computerised systems should be validated, applicable documentation revised and personnel trained, before the change is introduced into routine use. Computerised systems should be maintained in a validated state.

2.6   Donor session

General

Records should be kept for each activity associated with the donation. The record should reflect also any unsuccessful donation, the rejection of a donor, adverse reactions or unexpected events. An authorised interviewer should sign the donor selection records and final assessment.

The sterile blood bag systems should be used in accordance with the instructions of the manufacturer. A check should be made before use, to ensure that the collection system used is not damaged or contaminated, and that it is appropriate for the intended collection. Defects in blood bags should be reported to the supplier and subject to trend analysis.

The donor identification, donor selection interview and donor assessment should take place before each donation. The donor should be re-identified immediately prior to venipuncture.

Blood collection

For blood donations, laboratory samples should be taken at the time of donation. Procedures should be designed to minimise the risk of microbial contamination of the collected blood or deterioration of the sample, and to prevent potential misidentification of samples.

The venipuncture site should be prepared using a defined and validated disinfection procedure. The effectiveness of the disinfection procedure should be monitored and corrective action taken where indicated.

Where an anticoagulant solution is used in the collection, the collection bag should be mixed gently immediately after start of collection and at regular intervals thereafter during the whole collection period. The maximum collection time for acceptance of the donation for component processing should be specified and controlled. Donations that exceed the maximum time period should be recorded and discarded.

If integral blood bag collection tubing is to be used to prepare segments for testing, it should be sealed off at the end and then filled with anticoagulated blood as soon as possible after blood collection.

At completion of the donation, the donation number issued should be checked on all records, blood bags and laboratory samples. Donation number labels that have not been used should be destroyed via a controlled procedure. Routines to prevent misidentification should be in place.

After blood collection, the blood bags should be handled, transported and placed into storage according to defined procedures.

2.7 Processing

General

The procedures should detail the specifications for materials which will influence the quality of the final blood component. In particular, specifications should be in place for blood and blood components (intermediate and final components), starting material, additive solutions, primary package material (bags) and equipment.

Intermediate storage and transport

After collection, blood bags should be promptly placed into controlled temperature storage and transported to the processing site under temperature conditions appropriate for the component that will be prepared. There should be validation data to demonstrate that the storage after collection and method of transport maintains the blood within the specified temperature range throughout the period of transportation.

Processing of Blood Components

Time limits should be defined for the processing of blood components.

The premises used for the processing of blood components should be kept in a clean and hygienic condition and the microbial contamination load on critical equipment, surfaces and the environment of the processing areas should be monitored.

Sterile connecting devices should be used in accordance with a validated procedure. The resulting weld should be checked for satisfactory alignment and the integrity validated. If validated and used properly, connection done using sterile connecting devices can be regarded as closed system processing.

Irradiated components

Regular dose-mapping of gamma-irradiated equipment should be performed. The exposure time should be set to ensure that all blood and blood components receive the specified recommended minimum dose, with no part receiving more than the maximum recommended dose.

In case of a cobalt source, allowance should be made at least annually for source decay. A second independent timing device should be used to monitor exposure time.

Radiation indicators should be used as an aid to differentiating irradiated from non-irradiated blood and blood components. A defined procedure should ensure the segregation of components that have not been irradiated from those which have been irradiated.

Labelling

Before use all containers should be labelled with relevant information of their identity. The type of label to be used as well as the labelling methodology should be established in written procedures. Critical information should where possible be provided in machine readable format to eliminate transcription errors.

The blood establishment responsible for the processing of the blood component should supply the person(s) using the blood component with information on its use, composition, and special conditions that do not appear on the label.

Blood components for autologous use should be labelled as such.

Release of blood components

Each blood establishment should be able to demonstrate that a blood or blood component has been formally approved for release by an authorised person preferably assisted by validated information technology systems. The specifications for release of blood components must be defined, validated, documented and approved by QA.

There should be a system of administrative and physical quarantine for blood and blood components to ensure that they cannot be released until all mandatory requirements have been satisfied.

In the absence of a computerised system for product status control:

- the label of a blood component should identify the product status and should clearly distinguish released from non-released (quarantined) product;

- records should demonstrate that before a component is released, all current declaration forms, relevant medical records and test results have been verified by an authorised person.

Before final product release, if blood or blood component(s) have been prepared from a donor who has donated on previous occasions, a comparison with previous records should be made to ensure that current records accurately reflect the donor history.

Where release is subject to computer-derived information the following points should be checked:

- the computer system should be validated to be fully secure against the possibility of blood and blood components which do not fulfil all test or donor selecting criteria, being released;

- the manual entry of critical data, such as laboratory test results, should require independent verification by a second authorised person;

- there should be a hierarchy of permitted access to enter, amend, read or print data. Methods of preventing unauthorised entry should be in place, such as personal identity codes or passwords which are changed on a regular basis;

- the computer system should block the release of all blood or blood components considered not acceptable for release. There should also be a means to block the release of any future donation from the donor.

In the event that a final product fails release due to potential impact on patient safety all other implicated components should be identified and appropriate action should be taken. A check should be made to ensure that (if relevant) other components from the same donation(s) and components prepared from previous donations given by the donor(s) are identified. There should be an immediate update of the donor record(s) to ensure that the donor(s) cannot make a further donation, if appropriate.

2.8   Storage and distribution

General

Storage and distribution routines should take place in a safe and controlled way in order to assure product quality during the whole storage period and to exclude identification errors of blood components.
All transportation and storage actions, including receipt and distribution, should be defined by written procedures and specifications.

Storage

There should be a system in place to maintain and control the storage of blood components during their shelf life, including any transportation that may be required. Temperature and hygienic conditions should be monitored. Warning systems should be used where applicable. Autologous blood and blood components should be stored separately.

Distribution

Prior to distribution, blood components should be visually inspected. There should be a record identifying the person distributing and the customer receiving the components.

Blood components should not be returned for subsequent distribution, unless the procedure for return of a blood component is regulated by a contract and for each returned blood component it is proven that the agreed storage conditions have been met.

Before subsequent distribution the records should indicate that the blood component has been inspected before re-issue.

2.9   Quality monitoring

There should be data validating each process in the processing of blood and blood components to ensure that they meet specifications.

All critical processes should be validated.

There should also be quality control data demonstrating that the processes are in control. Acceptance criteria should be based on a defined set of specifications for each blood and blood component.

2.10   Quality control

General

All quality control procedures should be validated before use.

Quality control of blood and blood components should be carried out according to a defined sampling plan. The testing should be performed in accordance with the instructions recommended by the manufacturer of reagents and test kits.

The work record should identify the test(s) employed so as to ensure that entries, such as the calculation of results, are available for review.
The results of quality control testing should be subject to periodic review.

Quality control test results that do not satisfy the specified acceptance criteria should be clearly identified to ensure that blood and blood components of that donation remain in quarantine and the relevant samples are held for further testing.

The performance of the testing procedures should be regularly assessed by participation in a formal system of proficiency testing.

Screening tests for infectious disease markers

There should be clearly defined procedures to resolve discrepant results and to ensure that blood and blood components that have a repeatedly reactive result in a screening test for infectious markers shall be excluded from therapeutic use and be stored separately in a dedicated environment or destroyed. Appropriate confirmatory testing should take place. In case of confirmed positive results appropriate management of the donor should take place, including informing the donor and clear follow-up procedures.

Samples from each donation should be retained in frozen state to allow future testing.

When stored samples are tested, the test procedure must be validated for the specific storage conditions

Blood group serology testing

All first time donors should be tested for ABO and RhD blood groups and clinically significant irregular red cell antibodies. The ABO RhD labelling of the red cell concentrates of all first time donations should be based upon two independent ABO RhD tests.
Donors with a history of transfusions or pregnancy since the last donation should be tested for clinically significant irregular red cell antibodies. Where applicable, the blood or blood component should be labelled accordingly.

If the ABO and RhD blood group is verified on a subsequent donation, a comparison should be made of the historically determined blood group. If a discrepancy is found, the applicable blood components should not be released until the discrepancy is unequivocally resolved.

2.11 Contract management

If certain tasks, such as component processing or testing, are performed externally, these should be subject to a specific written contract. The contracting organisation should ensure that the contractor adheres to relevant good practice requirements.

2.12 Deviations, complaints, adverse events and reactions, recall, corrective and preventive actions

Deviations

There should be a defined procedure for the release of non-standard blood and blood components under a planned non-conformance system. The decision for such a release must be clearly documented and authorised by a designated person and traceability should be ensured.

Complaints, adverse events or reactions

There should be systems in place to ensure that complaints, adverse events or reactions are documented, carefully investigated for causative factors of the defect and, where necessary, followed by the implementation of corrective actions to prevent recurrence.

Recall of blood components

There should be a person within the blood establishment nominated to assess the need for product recall and to initiate and co-ordinate the necessary actions.

An effective recall procedure should be in place, including a description of the responsibilities and actions to be taken and guidance on the situations in which a recall may be required. Actions should be taken within pre-defined periods of time and should include tracing all relevant components and, where applicable, should include lookback procedures.

Corrective and preventive actions

All errors and accidents should be documented and investigated in order to identify system problems for correction. This includes 'near miss events'.

The corrective and preventive action system should ensure that existing product nonconformity or quality problems are corrected and that recurrence of the problem is prevented.

The blood establishment should have methods and procedures in place to input product or quality problems into the corrective and preventive action system.

Quality data should be routinely analysed to identify product and quality problems that may require corrective action or to identify unfavourable trends that may require preventive action.

2.13   Self inspection, audits and improvement

In order to monitor the implementation and compliance with the quality management system, systems of regular self-inspection and internal audits need to be in place. This should be conducted independently by trained and competent persons from within the organisation, according to approved protocols.

Inter-institutional audits should be actively promoted.
External inspections and audits by approved and competent authorities are necessary.

All audit results should be documented and reported to management. Appropriate corrective actions should be taken.

Preventive and corrective actions should be documented and assessed for effectiveness after implementation.

The management of a blood establishment should demonstrate a commitment towards continuous quality improvement. Input for this process can come from various sources such as complaints, errors, inspections, audits and suggestions.

PART B:
Blood collection

Chapter 1: Selection of donors

Principles of self-sufficiency from voluntary and non-remunerated donations have been recommended and promoted by the Council of Europe and have been defined in Article 2 of Council of Europe Recommendation No. R (95) 14 as follows:

> *"Donation is considered voluntary and non-remunerated if the person gives blood, plasma or cellular components of his/her own free will and receives no payment for it, either in the form of cash, or in kind which could be considered a substitute for money. This would include time off work other than that reasonably needed for the donation and travel. Small tokens, refreshments and reimbursements of direct travel costs are compatible with voluntary, non-remunerated donation."*

They have also been adopted by the Council of the European Communities in Directive 2002/98 EC which in the preamble (23) states: "The definition of voluntary and unpaid donation of the Council of Europe should be taken into account", and, in Article 20 paragraph 1: "Member States shall take the necessary measures to encourage voluntary and unpaid blood donations with a view to ensuring that blood and blood components are in so far as possible provided from such donations."

NB: *Specific immunisation programmes are not considered in this document but donors enrolled for this purpose should at least fulfil the minimum criteria outlined above (see also Annex 2, Requirements for the collection, processing and quality control of blood, blood components and plasma derivatives, WHO Technical Report Series, No. 840, 1994).*

Some criteria for the selection of donors vary according to the type of donation involved.

This chapter considers the selection of donors of whole blood and also donors of components obtained by different apheresis procedures. The selection of donors of haematopoietic progenitor cells is to be found in Chapter 2 of the "Guide to safety and quality assurance for organs, tissues and cells"(Council of Europe publications ISBN 92-871-4891-0).

There are general principles which apply to all donors. There are also further requirements specific to donors of different components collected by different methods.

This chapter is therefore divided into five sections:

A.   General principles of donor selection and guidelines for deferral;

B.   Considerations specific for donors of different types of components;

C.   Donor of red cells for anti D immunisation;

D.   Designated and directed donations;

E.   An example of a donor questionnaire.

A.   General principles of donor selection and guidelines for deferral

The main purpose of selecting individuals for blood and component donation is to determine whether the person is in good health, in order to safeguard both their health and the health of the recipient. All donors should undergo a screening process to assess their suitability.

Only healthy people with a good medical history should be accepted as donors of blood for therapeutic use.

Donor screening

A complete medical and physical examination of the donors is generally not possible in practice. One has to rely on the donor's appearance, their answers to simple questions concerning their medical history, general health, relevant lifestyle and simple laboratory tests.

Persons, whose sexual behaviour puts them at high risk of acquiring severe infectious diseases that can be transmitted by blood, should be permanently deferred.

The screening process involves:

- the provision of pre-donation educational material to all donors. This educational material should be understandable by the donors and explain the donation process, the transmission of blood borne infections and the donor's responsibility in preventing such transmission.

- an assessment of each donor carried out by a suitably qualified person, trained to use accepted guidelines and working under the direction of a physician. This assessment involves an interview, a questionnaire and further direct questions if necessary.

The questionnaire should be designed to elicit information relevant to the health and life style of the donor. It should be understandable by the donor and given to all donors each time they attend. On completion it should be signed by the donor and the person who carries out the assessment to certify that the relevant questions have been asked.

In order to obtain relevant and consistent information about the donor's medical history and general health, it is recommended that pre-printed questionnaires be completed, adapted to the type of donor (first time, regular, apheresis donor ,etc.).

An interview may be conducted with specifically trained staff who may ask further direct questions to supplement the information in the questionnaire. The interview should be conducted in privacy.

Deferred donors should be given a clear explanation of the reasons for deferral.

The main issues to be covered either by the questionnaire or by direct questions are included in an example questionnaire in section E.

Donor details

There must be secure, unique donor identification, contact details and robust audit trails linking donor to donation.

Age

Minimum: 18 years   Maximum: 65 years

- Where allowed, bleeding donors may be considered at the age of 17 in accordance with national legislation.

- Bleeding donors outside this age limit is at the discretion of the responsible physician, as is the recruitment of any first-time donor above the age of 60.

Hazardous occupations

Hazardous occupations or hobbies should normally entail an interval of not less than 12 hours between donation and returning to the occupation or hobby. Examples of such hazardous occupations or hobbies include piloting, bus or train driving, crane operating, climbing of ladders or scaffolding, gliding, climbing and diving.

Donor Appearance, Blood Pressure and Pulse

Special note should be taken of plethora, poor physique, debilitation, under-nutrition, anaemia, jaundice, cyanosis, dyspnoea, mental instability, intoxication from alcohol or drugs.

The skin at the venipuncture site should be free from lesions including local eczema.

Persons clearly under the influence of alcohol should be deferred until sober. Illicit parenteral drug taking if admitted or suspected must lead to permanent deferral.

If pulse and blood pressure is tested then the pulse should be regular and between 50 and 100 beats per minute. It is recognised that recording the blood pressure may be subject to several variables but as a guide the systolic blood pressure should not exceed 180 mm of mercury and the diastolic pressure 100 mm.

Guidelines for donor deferral

Based on the information obtained by the application of the questionnaire and interview the following guidelines should be followed. These are of necessity incomplete but encompass some of the main conditions.

Abnormal conditions should be referred to the physician in charge who has the responsibility of making the final decision. If the physician has any doubt about the donor's suitability they should be deferred.

Taking into account the requirement that only healthy people are acceptable as blood donors, deferral criteria are grouped into:

- Conditions requiring permanent deferral;
- Conditions requiring temporary deferral for defined time periods;
- Conditions requiring individual assessment;
- Infectious diseases.

Conditions leading to permanent deferral (rejection)

Cancer / Malignant Diseases	Individuals with a malignant disease, or a history of such, are usually permanently deferred. The physician in charge may make exceptions to this rule in selected cases. For example, donors may be accepted at the conclusion of successful treatment for non-invasive cervical cancer and rodent ulcer

Creutzfeldt-Jakob Disease	All individuals who have in the past been treated with extracts derived from human pituitary glands, have been recipients of dura mater or corneal grafts or who have been told of a family risk of Creutzfeldt-Jakob Disease or any other Transmissible Spongiform Encephalopathy*
Diabetes	If requiring insulin therapy
Drugs	Any history of injectable drug abuse
Heart and blood vessel disease	Persons with a history of heart disease, especially coronary disease, angina pectoris, severe cardiac arrhythmia, a history of cerebrovascular diseases, arterial thrombosis or recurrent venous thrombosis. (See also hypertension)
Infectious conditions	There are infectious states and diseases necessitating permanent deferral: Carriers of HIV 1/2, HTLV I/II, HBV, HCV Babesiosis† Leishmaniasis (Kala-Azar)† Chronic Q fever† Trypanosomiasis cruzi (Chagas disease)† Please see also section on Infectious diseases Persons, whose sexual behaviour puts them at high risk of acquiring severe infectious diseases that can be transmitted by blood
Xenotransplant recipients	Permanent deferral

---

* A family history of CJD carries a presumption of family risk unless it is determined that: (a) the affected family member had vCJD, not CJD; or (b) the affected family member did not have a genetic relationship to the donor; or (c) the cause of CJD in the affected family member was iatrogenic; or (d) the donor was tested and is known to have a normal genetic polymorphism for PrP^c.

† The tests and deferral periods indicated may be waived by the blood establishment when the donation is used exclusively for plasma for fractionation.

Conditions leading to temporary deferral (suspension)

Condition	Deferral period
Exposure to risk of acquiring a transfusion transmissible infection	
Endoscopy with biopsy using flexible instruments, inoculation injury, major surgery, acupuncture*, tattooing* or body piercing, mucosal splash with blood, tissue or cell transplant of human origin.	6 months or 4 months provided a NAT test for hepatitis C is negative.
Transfusion of blood components	6 months or for 4 months provided a NAT test for hepatitis C is negative. Injection of red cells as part of an approved immunisation programme will need clinical assessment.
Epilepsy	Three years off treatment and without an attack.
Fever above 38°C, flu-like illness	Two weeks following cessation of symptoms.
Kidney disease	Acute glomerulonephritis: five years deferral period following complete recovery.
Medication	The taking of a medication may indicate an underlying disease which may disqualify the donor. It is recommended that a list of commonly used drugs, with rules for acceptability of donors, approved by the medical staff of the transfusion centre, be available. Donors treated with prescribed drugs, particularly those with proven teratogenic effect, should be deferred for a period consistent with the pharmacokinetic properties of the drug.
Osteomyelitis	Two years after having been declared cured.
Pregnancy	6 months after delivery or termination, except in exceptional circumstances and at the discretion of a physician.
Rheumatic fever	Two years following attack with no evidence of chronic heart disease. The latter complication is a cause for permanent deferral.

---

*   Exceptions could be made according to national risk assessment.

Condition	Deferral period
Surgery	Following major surgery patients should not donate until they are fully recovered and fit to be donors, typically about six months.
Tooth extraction	If no complications, one week (because of possible risk of transient bacteraemia).
Tropical Diseases	6 months following return from tropical areas and then only if they have not suffered an unexplained fever or illness (see infectious diseases).

Prophylactic immunisations

Inoculations, vaccinations	Deferral period
1. Vaccines with attenuated bacteria and viruses: BCG, yellow fever, rubella, measles, poliomyelitis (oral) mumps, live attenuated typhoid fever vaccine, live attenuated cholera vaccine	Four weeks
2. Vaccines with killed bacteria Cholera, typhoid, Capsular polysaccharide typhoid fever vaccine	Accept if well
3. Vaccines with inactivated viruses Poliomyelitis (injection), influenza	Accept if well
4. Toxoids Diphtheria, tetanus	Accept if well
5. Other vaccines Hepatitis A vaccine Hepatitis B vaccine	Accept if well and no exposure (see section on jaundice and hepatitis)
Rabies, tick-borne encephalitis	Accept if well One year if post-exposure

Conditions requiring individual assessment

As donors may present with a variety of medical problems, past or present only some of the more common examples are considered here.

It is recommended that national authorities develop detailed guidance based on prevailing conditions in the populations they serve.

Allergy	Individuals with a documented history of anaphylaxis should not be accepted as donors.
Auto-immune diseases	If more than one organ is affected this leads to permanent deferral.
Beta thalassaemia trait	Heterozygote carriers of beta-thalassaemia trait may give blood provided they are in good health and have a haemoglobin level within acceptable values.
Bronchitis	Persons with symptoms of severe chronic bronchitis should not be accepted as donors.
Common cold	Accept, if asymptomatic and feels well on the day of donation.
Hypertension	A person who presents with a systolic blood pressure of more than 180 mm Hg or a diastolic blood pressure of more than 100 mm Hg should not be accepted as a blood donor. A mild hypertensive whose diastolic blood pressure is maintained at less than 100 mm Hg may be accepted.

Infectious diseases

Following infectious diseases generally a deferral period of at least two weeks after cessation of symptoms should be respected.

If there was contact with an infectious disease, the deferral period should equal the incubation period, or if unknown, the nature of the contact and the deferral period has to be determined by the responsible physician.

Some emerging infectious diseases may represent a threat to the safety of blood transfusion. A risk / benefit analysis should be carried out on a country by country basis. Precautionary measures, which should be proportionate to the risk, should be implemented in a timely fashion in line with the emerging evidence. Donor selection policies to address the risk may include deferral for a suitable period of donors exposed in geographic areas where the disease is occurring. The introduction of appropriate testing strategies may have to be considered.

Reported cases of post transfusion infections should be investigated by appropriate lookback studies.

a)   *Acquired Immune Deficiency Syndrome (AIDS) HIV infection*

All blood donors should be provided with accurate and updated information on HIV transmission and AIDS so that those persons who have unsafe sex practices or other risk behaviour exposing them to potential infectious sources will refrain from donating. The information provided may vary between countries according to local epidemiological data. Blood and blood products with a repeat positive marker for HIV should not be used for therapeutic purposes. All blood donors found to have a confirmed positive marker for HIV should be informed, as part of a full counselling procedure, that they should not give further donations. Donors found to have a repeat positive marker for HIV which cannot be confirmed should be informed according to the nationally agreed algorithm.

Sexual partners:

- current sexual partners of people with HIV should be deferred;
- previous sexual partners of people with HIV are acceptable after 12 months since the last sexual contact.

b)   *Brucellosis (confirmed)*

Deferral for at least two years following full recovery.

The test and the deferral period may be waived by the blood establishment when the donation is used exclusively for plasma fractionation.

c)   *Chagas disease*

Individuals with Chagas disease or who have had Chagas disease should be deferred permanently.

The blood of persons who were born or have been transfused in areas where the disease is endemic should be used only for plasma fractionation products unless a validated test for infection with *T. cruzi* is negative.

d)   *Jaundice and Hepatitis*

Donors should be provided with up-to-date information on the risk activities which may be associated with hepatitis transmission to provide the opportunity for self-exclusion. Individuals with a history of jaundice or hepatitis may, at the discretion of the appropriate competent medical authority, be accepted as blood donors provided an approved test for HBsAg and anti HCV is negative. Persons whose blood gives a positive reaction for the presence of HBsAg and/or anti HCV are excluded.

It should be noted that following hepatitis B immunisation, a transient positive HBsAg result may be obtained.

The presence of anti-HBs does not lead to deferral.

Persons who have been in close household contact with a case of hepatitis B infection (acute or chronic) should be deferred for six months from the time of contact unless demonstrated to be immune.

Hospital staff coming into direct contact with patients with hepatitis are accepted at the discretion of the physician in charge of the blood-collecting unit providing they have not suffered an inoculation injury or mucous membrane exposure, in which case they should be deferred for six months.

Sexual partners:

- current sexual partners of people with HBV should be deferred unless demonstrated to be immune;
- previous sexual partners of people with HBV are acceptable after 6 months since the last sexual contact.

e) *Malaria**

Donors of blood components
(Whole blood, red cells, platelets, or plasma for direct clinical transfusion)

Since questioning the donor as to the country(s) in which he was born, brought up or has visited is essential for effective detection, every transfusion service should have a current map of the endemic zones and an alphabetical list of the countries concerned.

Persons who have lived in a malaria area for a continuous period of 6 months or more at any time in life

These persons may become symptomless carriers of the malaria parasite. Therefore, the following rules must apply to these individuals after each return from a malaria area.

- May be accepted as blood donor if the result of a validated immunological test for antibodies to the malaria parasite, taken at least 4 months after the last visit to a malaria area is negative.
- If the test is positive the donor should be permanently deferred.
- If a test is not performed the donor should be permanently deferred.

---

*   The test and the deferral periods may be waived by the blood establishment when the donation is used exclusively for plasma fractionation.

Persons who give a history of malaria

- Should be deferred until asymptomatic and off treatment.

- May be accepted as blood donor if the result of a validated immunological test for antibodies to the malaria parasite, taken *at least 4 months* since cessation of treatment/last symptoms is negative.

- If the test is positive the donor should be deferred and may be re-evaluated after 3 years.

- If a test is not performed the donor should be permanently deferred.

Persons who report an undiagnosed febrile illness consistent with malaria during or within 6 months of the end of a visit to a malaria area:

- May be accepted as blood donor if the result of a validated immunological test for antibodies to the malaria parasite.

- Taken at least 4 months since cessation of treatment/last symptoms is negative.

- It the test is positive the donor should be deferred and may be re-evaluated after 3 years.

- If a test is not performed the donor should be deferred for 3 years.

All other persons who have visited a malaria endemic area

- May be accepted as a blood donors if the result of a validated immunological test for antibodies to the malaria parasite is negative, on a sample take at least 4 months after the last visit to a malaria endemic area.

- If the test is positive the donor should be deferred and be re-evaluated after 3 years.

- If a test is not performed, the donor may be re-accepted once a period of 12 months has elapsed after last return from a malaria area.

Donors of plasma for fractionation

The deferral periods and test regimes mentioned above may be omitted for those donors who give plasma that is used exclusively for fractionation into plasma derivatives.

f)   Q Fever∗

May be accepted two years after having been declared cured.

g)   Syphilis∗

May be accepted one year after having been declared cured.

h)   Toxoplasmosis

Deferral for six months following clinical recovery.

i)   Tuberculosis

May be accepted two years after having been declared cured.

j)   Variant Creutzfeldt-Jakob Disease

A new variant of Creutzfeldt-Jakob Disease (vCJD) has been described. It is accepted that BSE and vCJD are caused by the same agent.

Transfusion transmission of a variety of TSE agents has been demonstrated in animal models, and a case of human transfusion transmission by vCJD has been reported.

The Council of Europe, in its Recommendation N° R(2001)4 on the prevention of the possible transmission of variant Creutzfeldt-Jakob disease (vCJD) by blood transfusion has recommended various initiatives to minimise the risk of transmission of this agent by transfusion.

These recommendations suggest that the precautionary measures taken by countries take account of both the endogenous exposure of the population to bovine products from countries with a high BSE prevalence and the incidence of vCJD in the population. Any proposed precautionary measures should also take account of the impact on donors and the availability of blood and blood components.

Some measures currently taken by different countries include: leukocyte depletion; deferral of donors for geographical reasons; exclusion of donors transfused with components; decreasing the donor exposure for recipients; non-use of indigenous plasma for fractionation.

It is important that such measures should always be based on appropriate risk assessment. Increased attention should be given to the appropriate clinical use of blood and blood products.

∗   The tests and deferral periods may be waived by the blood establishment when the donation is used exclusively for plasma fractionation.

k) *West Nile Virus*

May be accepted 28 days after leaving an area with on-going transmission to humans of the disease.

B. Specific considerations for donors of different types of components

Whole Blood Donors

A standard donation should not be collected from persons weighing less than 50 kg.

Interval between donations

It is acknowledged that current practices in some transfusion services in Europe allow up to six standard donations per year to be taken from males and up to four per year from females, with a minimum interval between standard donations of two months.

It is recommended that these donation rates never be exceeded under any circumstances, and be accepted by any transfusion service only after careful consideration of the dietary habits of the populations concerned, and in the knowledge that extra care may be necessary, beyond routine haemoglobin or haematocrit estimation, in the monitoring of donors for iron deficiency. It is further recommended that an active donor panel be maintained of sufficient size to allow donors to be bled less often than the maximum rates stated, with the recommendation that four donations for males and three donations for females should ordinarily not be exceeded, thus affording the donors extra protection and giving the system flexibility to deal with large-scale emergency situations.

Quantity of donation

A standard donation is 450 ml ± 10% exclusive of anticoagulants. It is acknowledged that current practices in some transfusion services in Europe allow 500 ml ± 10% as a standard donation. No more than 13% of the estimated blood volume should be taken as whole blood during one blood donation. The blood volume may be estimated from sex/height and weight of the donor.

Laboratory examination:

- Haemoglobin or haematocrit (Hct.): should be determined each time the donor attends to donate.
- Minimum values before donation:
    - female donors: 125 g/l or 7.8 mmol/l (min. Hct = 0.38);
    - male donors: 135 g/l or 8.4 mmol/l (min. Hct = 0.4).

- Individual donations may be accepted below these levels after consultation with the responsible physicians or as established by a national control authority based on norms for their specific populations.

- It is recognised that blood donation may result in iron deficiency in repeat blood donors. This problem may arise without being evident through pre-donation haemoglobin measurement. This may be especially important in women in the child-bearing years. Blood establishments should include appropriate measures to minimise this problem, and to protect donor health. Such measures may include the use of tests to assess iron status, the provision of materials for donor education particularly in regard to the importance of an iron rich diet, the tailoring of donation frequency based on iron status and if appropriate the supplementation of a dietary iron through appropriate prophylactic medication. At the same time, blood establishments should recognise that many donors currently deferred because of low haemoglobin are in a satisfactory state of health and, once their iron status is confirmed as satisfactory, they may be re-entered into donation programs. Therefore, managing the problem of iron-deficiency contributes to the maintenance of donor health and the sufficiency of the blood supply.

- Abnormally high and low values should be further investigated, as should a fall in haemoglobin concentration of more than 20 g/litre between two successive donations.

Apheresis donors

The supervision and medical care of apheresis donors should be the responsibility of a physician specially trained in these techniques.

Other than in exceptional circumstances (to be decided by the responsible physician), donors for apheresis procedures shall meet the criteria for ordinary whole blood donations.

People with sickle cell trait should not be submitted to apheresis procedures.

Special attention should be given to the following conditions:

- abnormal bleeding episodes;

- a history suggestive of fluid retention (of special interest if steroids and/or plasma expanders are to be used);

- the taking of drugs containing acetylsalicylic acid within five days prior to thrombocytapheresis;

- a history of gastric symptoms (if steroids are to be used);

- adverse reactions to previous donations.

Frequency of donation and maximal amounts of removal of plasma and red cells

The following recommendations are made in the absence of conclusive studies of outcomes from different regimes of volumes and frequencies of plasmapheresis.

Donors should not be subjected to plasmapheresis more often than once every 2 weeks. Under exceptional circumstances and at the discretion of the responsible physician this frequency may be exceeded but the following guidelines on maximum volumes removed should be followed:

- Not more than 15 litres of plasma should be removed from one donor per year;

- Not more than 1 litre of plasma should be removed from one donor per week;

- In the absence of volume replacement, not more than 600 ml net volume of donor plasma should be removed from one donor per apheresis procedure. The net volume of donor plasma removed can either be calculated by subtracting the actual amount of anticoagulant in the collection bag(s) from the total volume of anticoagulated plasma in the bags, or can be approximated by respecting an upper limit of 650 ml of anticoagulated plasma to be collected. A suitable form of fluid replacement should be provided if the plasma plus anticoagulant volume withdrawn in one session exceeds 650 ml;

- When combining the collection of plasma, platelets, and/or red cells in one apheresis procedure, the total net volume of donor plasma, platelets and red cells should not exceed 600 ml. A suitable form of fluid replacement should be provided if the net volume removed from the donor in one session exceeds 600 ml;

- The total amount of red cells should not exceed the theoretical amount of red cells that would bring the donor haemoglobin in isovolemic situation below 110 g/l* or 6.8 mmol/l;

- The interval between one plasmapheresis or plateletpheresis procedure and a whole blood donation or single unit red cell apheresis (combined or not with plasma and/or platelet collection)

---

*   Calculated according to the following equation:
Estimated Post Hb = (TBV x pre Hb − amount Hb removed) / TBV
Where:
TBV = estimated donor total blood volume;
Amount Hb removed = includes red cells collected plus samples taken and red cells in the apheresis set not returned to the donor under normal circumstances.

should be at least 48 hours. The interval between a whole blood donation, an apheresis red cell collection or failed return of red cells during apheresis, and the next apheresis procedure without red cell collection, should be at least one month. The interval between two single unit red cell collections should be the same as for whole blood collections;

- The interval between whole blood donation and the donation of 2 units of red cells should be at least 3 months. The interval between a 2 unit red cell apheresis and whole blood donation or another 2 unit red cell apheresis should be at least 6 months. Total erythrocyte loss/year should not exceed that acceptable for whole blood donors;

- For autologous 2 unit red cell apheresis shorter time limits may be accepted at the discretion of the responsible physician.

Additional requirements for donors undergoing plasmapheresis

- Protein analysis, such as determination of total serum or plasma protein and/or electrophoresis and/or quantitation of single proteins, especially albumin and IgG; total proteins should not be less than 60 g/l. This analysis should be carried out at suitable intervals but at least annually.

Donors undergoing plasmapheresis more frequently than once every two weeks the following should be carried out at suitable intervals and at least annually:

- Evaluation by a physician of the total serum or plasma protein values and/or electrophoresis and/or quantitation of single proteins, especially albumin and IgG. Special attention should be paid to any significant fall in these values even though they may still come within the accepted normal limits.

Additional requirements for donors undergoing cytapheresis

- Requirements for thrombocytapheresis: platelet count-routine thrombocytapheresis should not be carried out on individuals whose normal count is less than 150×10^9 per litre;

- For routine provision of platelets by apheresis, an individual should not be subjected to the procedure more than once every two weeks. In the case of specific HLA/HPA cytapheresis, the interval may be reduced at the discretion of the physician responsible for the procedure.

Requirements for 1 unit red cell apheresis
(alone or combined with plasma and/or platelets)

- Haemoglobin or haematocrit should be examined before donation and should conform to those specified for whole blood donation;

- The total collected volume of the red cell unit should be subtracted from the total volume of plasma that can be collected in combined procedures with platelet and/or plasma collections. The same restrictions apply for the plasma and platelet portion of the procedure as for those procedures without red cell collection.

Requirements for 2 unit red cell apheresis

- The donor should have an estimated blood volume of > 5L (a requirement generally met by a non-obese person weighing > 70 kg);

- Haemoglobin should be examined before donation and the minimum value should be >140 g/L or 8.7 mmol/L (minimal haematocrit > 0.42). For the safety of the donor the haemoglobin level should not fall below 110g/L or 6.8 mmol/L after donation;

- For autologous 2 unit red cell apheresis lower haemoglobin levels can be accepted at the discretion of the responsible physician.

C.   Red cell donors for anti D immunisation

This section does not consider specific immunisation programmes but red cell donors enrolled for this purpose should at least fulfil the following minimum criteria:

- Infectious markers to be performed include HBsAg and antibodies to HIV-1/2, HCV, HTLV-I/II, HBc, and NAT test for proviral HIV-DNA and HCV-RNA. HBV-DNA in plasma should be considered;

- An extensive red cells phenotyping should be performed at least twice;

- The red cells for immunisation should be stored for at least 6 months. After 6 months all the above stated infectious markers should be found negative on a new donor sample before release of the stored red cells for immunisation;

- To address changes in donor selection criteria and infectious marker testing for regular whole blood donations that may occur over time, immunisation programs should:

a)   maintain retention samples from each RBC donation suitable for future testing;

b)   requalify past donations by current screening and testing of the donor whenever feasible or, testing of retention samples when current donor screening and testing is infeasible or insufficient to exclude a prior risk;

c)   exempt prior collections of RBCs from current standards only after careful considerations of the risks to the immunised donors and ultimate plasma product recipients.

D.   Designated and directed donations

Although blood donation is voluntary, non-remunerated and anonymous, in some special circumstances it may be necessary to make use of designated donations. This should happen only for clear medical indications.

Designated donations

Designated donations are those intended for named patients based on medical indications. These donations may include family members, but clinical benefits for the patient are weighed against the risk by the physician. Circumstances where this may occur are:

1.   for patients with rare blood types, where no compatible anonymous donations are available;

2.   in case donor-specific transfusions are indicated for immune modulation or immunotherapy, for instance in the preparation procedure for kidney transplant or for lymphocyte transfusions aimed at a graft-versus-leukaemia effect;

3.   in certain cases of alloimmune neonatal thrombocytopenia, for instance, when HPA typed platelets are not available and IVIG therapy is insufficient.

The practice of transfusing parental blood to infants is not without risk. Mothers may have antibodies to antigens which are present on the infant's red blood cells, platelets or white blood cells, therefore maternal plasma should not be transfused. Fathers should not serve as cell donors to neonates, because maternal antibodies to antigens inherited from the father may have been transmitted through the placenta to the foetus. In addition due to partial histocompatibility, transfusions of cells from parental or family donors carry an increased risk of GVHD, even in the immunocompetent.

Directed donations

Directed donations are those intended for named patients, where the request for the donation has been made by patients, relatives, or friends. The public often believes directed donations to be safer than anonymous voluntary non-remunerated donations, but this is not the case, and infectious disease marker rates are in general higher among directed donors.

Directed donations are not considered good practice and should be discouraged.

E.   An example of a donor questionnaire

General questions

- Are you in good health?

- For women: Have you had a pregnancy in the past year?

- Do you have a hazardous occupation or hobby?

- Have you previously been told not to give blood?

- Have you experienced any unexplained fever?

- Are you currently on any medication, including aspirin?

- Have you had any recent vaccinations or dental treatment?

- Have you ever had medication with isotretinoin (e.g.: Accutane R), etretinate (e.g.: Tegison R), acitretin (e.g.: Neotigason R) finasteride (e.g.: Proscar R, Propecia R,), dutasteride (e.g. Avodart R)?

- Have you ever suffered from any serious illness such as:

    - jaundice, malaria, tuberculosis, rheumatic fever?

    - heart disease, high or low blood pressure?

    - severe allergy, asthma?

    - convulsions or diseases of the nervous system?

    - chronic diseases such as diabetes or malignancies?

Questions related to HIV /HBV /HCV infection risk

- Have you read and understood the information on AIDS (HIV infection) and hepatitis?

- Have you ever injected any drugs?

- Have you ever accepted payment for sex in money or drugs?

- For men: have you ever had sex with another man?

- For women: to the best of your knowledge has any man with whom you have had sex in the past 12 months had sex with a man?

- During the past 12 months have you had sexual contact with someone who:

    - is HIV positive or has hepatitis?

    - has injected drugs?

    - receives or has received payment for sex in money or drugs?

- Have you had a sexually transmitted disease?

- Have you been exposed to hepatitis? (family or job)?

- Since your last donation or in the previous 12 months have you had:

    - an operation or medical investigations?

    - any body piercing and /or tattoo?

    - acupuncture treatment by anyone other than a registered practitioner?

    - a transfusion?

    - an accidental injury involving a needle and /or mucous membrane exposure to blood?

Questions related to CJD risk

- Have you been told of a family history of Creutzfeldt-Jakob Disease (CJD)?

- Have you had a corneal graft?

- Have you ever had a dura mater graft?

- Have you ever had treatment with human pituitary extracts?

Questions related to travel risk

- Were you born or have you lived and/or travelled abroad? where?

Chapter 2: Blood collection

1.   Premises for donor sessions

When sessions are performed by mobile teams, a realistic attitude towards environmental standards is necessary. The premises should satisfy common sense requirements for the health and safety of both the mobile teams and the donors concerned, with due regard to relevant legislation or regulations. Points to check should include adequate heating, lighting and ventilation, general cleanliness, provision of a secure supply of water and electricity, adequate sanitation, compliance with fire regulations, satisfactory access for unloading and loading of equipment by the mobile team, adequate space to allow free access to the bleed, and rest beds. Facilities should be provided for a confidential interview with each donor.

When the sessional venue is permanent and under the control of the transfusion centre, provision should additionally be made for proper cleaning by, for example, the use of non-slip, washable floor material installed without inaccessible corners, avoidance of internal window ledges, etc. Where possible, ventilation should be by an air-conditioning unit to avoid the need for open windows. Air changes, together with temperature and humidity control, should be adequate to cope with the maximum number of people likely to be in the room, and with the heat output from any equipment used. A maximum/minimum thermometer should be installed and checked daily.

2.   Equipment used at blood donation sessions

Reference should be made to Chapter 24 for quality control procedures to be applied to equipment used at blood donation sessions.

The manufacturer's label on the blood containers (blood plastic bags and bag systems) should contain the following eye readable information: the manufacturer's name and address, the name of the blood bag and/or the name of the blood bag plastic material, the name, composition and volume of anticoagulant or additive solution (if any), the product catalogue number and the lot number. It is recommended that the manufacturer's identity and container information (catalogue number and the container number of the set) as well as the manufacturer's lot number should be given in eye and machine readable codes.

3.   **Pre-donation checks and labelling**

- The blood containers should be inspected before use for defects as well as after the donation. Defects may be hidden behind the label pasted on the container. The container should be inspected before use for the prescribed content (and appearance) of the anticoagulant solution. Abnormal moisture or discolouration on the surface of the bag or label after unpacking suggests leakage through a defect. If one or more bags in any package is found to be abnormally damp all the bags in the package should be rejected.

- At the time of the blood donation, the blood container as well as those of the samples collected for testing should be labelled to uniquely identify the blood donation. The labelling system should comply with the relevant national legislation and international agreements. The blood donation should be identified by a unique identity number which is both eye and machine readable. The unique identity number may consist of a code for the responsible blood collection organisation, the year of donation and a serial number. The labelling system should allow full traceability to all relevant data registered by the blood establishment about the donor and the blood donation.

- Careful check must be made of the identity of the donor against the labels issued for that donation.

4.   **Preparation of the phlebotomy site**

Although it is impossible to guarantee 100% sterility of the skin surface for phlebotomy, a strict, standardised procedure for the preparation of the phlebotomy area should exist. Of particular importance is that the antiseptic solution used be allowed to dry completely before venipuncture, The time taken will vary with the product used but should be subject to an absolute minimum of 30 seconds. The prepared area must not be touched with fingers before the needle has been inserted.

5.   **Need for successful venipuncture and proper mixing**

The bleeding should be carried out in the following manner:

a)   The needle should be inserted into the vein at first attempt. A second clean venipuncture with a new needle at a separate site is acceptable.

b)   Proper mixing of the blood with the anti-coagulant should be guaranteed at all phases of the bleeding. To achieve this, one should pay attention to the following details:

- as the blood begins to flow, it must immediately come into contact with the anticoagulant and properly mixed;

- the flow of the blood must be sufficient and uninterrupted. Donation of a whole blood unit should ideally not last more than 10 minutes. If duration of the bleeding is longer than 12 minutes, the blood should not be used for the preparation of platelets. If the duration of the bleeding is longer than 15 minutes, the plasma should not be used for direct transfusion or the preparation of coagulation factors;

- in the case of apheresis, any interruption of the flow occurring during the procedure should exclude that donation from fractionation of labile plasma proteins or for the preparation of platelets;

- when manual mixing is used, the blood bag must be inverted every 30-45 seconds. When an automated mixing is used, an appropriately validated system is required.

6.   Handling of filled containers and samples

Plastic containers should be checked after donation for any defect. During separation from the donor of the freshly filled plastic bag of blood, a completely efficient method of sealing the tube is obligatory.

Immediately after sealing of the collection bag, the contents of the bag line should be completely discharged into the bag. The test samples should be taken directly from the bleed line or the sample pouch of the collection system.

The organisation should be such as to minimise the possibility of errors in labelling of blood containers and blood samples. In this respect, it is recommended that each bed should have its individual facilities for the handling of samples during donation and labelling. Taking of samples at the end of donation should be directly linked with the cessation of donation with the minimum possible time interval. The blood bag and corresponding samples should not be removed from the donor's bedside until a satisfactory check on correct labelling has been carried out.

7.   Special requirements for apheresis

Separation and collection of blood components by cell-separators requires premises of suitable size, regular service and maintenance of the machines, and adequately trained personnel for operating such machines.

The donor should be observed closely during the procedure and a physician familiar with all aspects of apheresis must be available in order to provide assistance and emergency medical care procedures in case of adverse reaction.

Routine premedication of donors for the purpose of increasing component yield is not recommended.

The volume of extracorporeal blood should not exceed 13% of the donor's estimated blood volume.

8. Return of red blood cells of donors undergoing manual apheresis

Since the biggest inherent danger in manual apheresis is an interchange between two bags of concentrated red blood cells during their centrifugation and return to individual donors, a proper identification system to avoid this is an absolute necessity. For instance the donor may be asked to sign the label of the bag and to confirm his signature before the return of the red cells, though the ultimate responsibility lies with the individual carrying out this procedure.

In addition, use can be made of the integral numbering system on the pilot tube of plastic bags, perhaps by transferring this number to the wrist of the donor.

9. Storage of donor samples

The retention of donor samples for a period of time may provide useful information. The provision of such systems is contingent on the availability of adequate human and financial resources.

10. Donor clinic documentation

Full records must be maintained at blood donation sessions, to cover the following parameters:

i.   the date, donation number, identity, and medical history of the donor;

ii.   the date, donation number, identity, and medical history of the donor for each unsuccessful donation, with reasons for the failure of the donation;

iii. list of rejected donors with the reasons for their rejection;

iv.   full details of any adverse reactions in a donor at any stage of the procedure;

v.   for apheresis donor: volume of collection, volume of blood processed, volume of replacement solution and volume of anticoagulant.

As far as possible the records of blood donation sessions should allow identification by blood transfusion staff of each important phase associated with the donation. These records should be used for the regular compilation of statistics which should be studied by the individual with ultimate responsibility for the blood donation session, who will take such action on them as deemed necessary.

Chapter 3: Principles of component preparation

1. Blood components - why should they be used?

Transfusion therapy in the past was largely dependent on the use of whole blood. While whole blood may still be used in certain limited circumstances, the thrust of modern transfusion therapy is to use the specific component that is clinically indicated. Components are those therapeutic constituents of blood that can be prepared by centrifugation, filtration and freezing using conventional blood bank methodology.

Transfusions are used mainly for the following purposes:

- to maintain oxygen/carbon dioxide transport
- to correct bleeding and coagulation disorders

It is evident that one single product, whole blood, is not necessarily suitable for all these purposes unless the patient requiring treatment has multiple deficiencies. Even then, the storage defects of whole blood make it unsuitable for such replacement. Patients should be given the component needed to correct their specific deficiency. This will avoid unnecessary and possibly harmful infusion of surplus constituents. The change from collection of blood in glass bottles to multiple plastic bag systems has greatly facilitated the preparation of high quality components. Storage considerations are a major reason for promoting the use of components. Optimal conditions and consequently shelf life vary for different components. Red cells maintain functional capability best when refrigerated. The quality of plasma constituents is best maintained in the frozen state while platelet storage is at room temperature with continuous agitation. Thus it is only the red cells whose storage requirement is fulfilled when whole blood is stored refrigerated, with consequent loss of therapeutic effectiveness of most of the other constituents.

Component therapy also offers logistic, ethical and economic advantages. The majority of patients requiring transfusion do not need the plasma in the whole unit and certainly not at a 1 to 1 ratio. Production of plasma derived products can thus be facilitated by the use of red cells rather than whole blood. Leukocyte depletion may further improve the quality of blood components.

2.   Preparation procedure

Blood components may be prepared during collection using apheresis technology. Plasma, leukocytes, platelets and red cell concentrates may be obtained thus. Alternatively, whole blood may be collected in the traditional manner with the components being made available by the post-donation processing of whole blood.

Due to the potential deterioration of activity and function of labile blood components, conditions of storage and time prior to processing are vital to the preparation of components. Delays in preparation or unsuitable conditions of storage may adversely affect quality of the final products.

3.   Choice of anticoagulant and bag system

Whole blood is collected into a bag containing an anticoagulant solution. The solution contains citrate and cell nutrients such as glucose and adenine. The first centrifugation steps will remove more than half of these nutrients from the residual red cells. Thus it may be more logical to provide the proper nutrients for the cells using a resuspension medium instead of incorporating them in the initial anticoagulant solution.

Plasticware used for blood collection, apheresis and component preparation should comply with the requirements of the relevant supplement of the European Pharmacopoeia with regard to haemocompatibility in addition to its suitability for achieving the respective technological goal. Polyvinyl chloride (PVC) has been found satisfactory for red blood cell storage. The biocompatibility of any plasticisers used must be assured. Storage of platelets at + 20 °C to + 24 °C requires a plastic with increased oxygen permeability. This has been achieved by plastic materials of alternative physical and/or chemical characteristics. Leaching of plasticisers into blood or a component should not pose any undue risk to the recipient. Any possible leaching of adhesives from labels or other device components should be kept within acceptable safety limits. Care should be taken to minimise levels of residual toxic substances after sterilisation, for example ethylene oxide.

Whenever new plastics are to be introduced an adequate study of component preparation and/or storage should be conducted. The following parameters could be useful:

- red blood cells: glucose, pH, haematocrit, haemolysis, ATP, lactate, extracellular potassium and 2,3-bisphosphoglycerate;

- platelets: pH, pO_2, pCO_2, bicarbonate ion, glucose, lactate accumulation, ATP, LDH release, beta thromboglobulin release, response from hypotonic shock and swirling phenomenon;

- plasma: Factor VIII and signs of coagulation activation, for example thrombin - antithrombin complexes.

These studies would normally be carried out by the manufacturer before introduction of the new plasticware and the results be made available to the transfusion services.

The evaluation of new plasticware can be completed by the evaluation of 24 hours post transfusion in vivo recovery and survival of autologous red cells and by the assessment of platelet recovery, survival and corrected count increments (CCI).

In order to maintain a closed system throughout the separation procedure, a multiple bag configuration, either ready made or sterile-docked, should be used. The design and arrangement of the pack system should be such as to permit the required sterile preparation of the desired component.

Although only use of closed systems is recommended for all steps in component processing, open systems may sometimes be necessary due to local constraints in an environment specifically designed to minimise the risk of bacterial contamination. When open systems are employed, careful attention should be given to use of aseptic procedures. The red cells so prepared should be transfused within 24 hours of processing. The platelets so prepared should be transfused within 6 hours of processing.

4.   Principles of centrifugation

The sedimentation behaviour of blood cells is determined by their size as well as the difference of their density from that of the surrounding fluid (see Table 3(a)). Other factors are viscosity of the medium and flexibility of the cells which are temperature dependent. The optimal temperature with respect to these factors is +20°C or higher.

Table 3(a):   Volume and density of principal blood constituents

	Mean Density (g/ml)	Mean Volume (10^{-15} litre)
Plasma	1.026	
Platelets	1.058	9
Monocytes	1.062	470
Lymphocytes	1.070	230
Neutrophils	1.082	450
Red Cells	1.100	87

In the first phase of centrifugation, the surrounding fluid is only a mixture of plasma and anticoagulant solution. Leukocytes and red cells now sediment more rapidly than platelets as they both have a bigger volume than platelets.

In a later phase, depending on the time and speed of centrifugation, most of the leukocytes and red cells therefore settle in the lower half of the bag and the upper half contains platelet rich plasma. More prolonged centrifugation results in platelet sedimentation driven by a force proportional to the square of the number of rotations per minute and the distance of each cell to the centre of the rotor, whereas the leukocytes being now surrounded by a fluid of higher density (the red cell mass), move upwards. At the end of centrifugation, cell-free plasma is in the upper part of the bag and red cells at the bottom.

Platelets accumulate on top of the red cell layer, while the majority of leukocytes are to be found immediately below in the top 10 ml of red cell mass. Haematopoietic progenitor cells have similar characteristics to normal mononuclear blood cells. However, their contaminants may be immature or malignant cells from different haematopoietic lineages which commonly have larger sizes and lower densities than their mature counterparts.

The choice to be made is the speed and time of centrifugation which will determine the composition of the desired component, i.e. if platelet-rich plasma is desired, centrifugation should stop prior to the phase where platelet sedimentation commences. A low centrifugation speed will allow for some variation in centrifugation time. If cell-free plasma is required, fast centrifugation for an adequate time will allow separation to cell-poor plasma and densely packed cells. It is important that the optimal conditions for a good separation be carefully standardised for each centrifuge. A number of choices exist for the selection of a procedure for centrifugation for component preparation from whole blood.

Table 3(b) outlines five different methods of performing the first step in the separation of whole blood as well as the approximate composition of the resulting initial components. The choice of the initial separation step strongly influences the methods of further processing of the initial fractions. This leads to a system of interdependent preparation of a blood component is specified, reference should always be made to the initial separation step.

5.   Separation

5.1.   Separation after the initial centrifugation

After centrifugation, the bag system is carefully removed from the centrifuge. The primary bag is placed into a plasma extraction system and the layers are transferred, one by one, into satellite bags within the closed system.

The choice to be made is whether or not the buffy coat is to be separated from the packed cells. The advantage of this is that the red cells are leukocyte-poor and will remain aggregate-poor during storage. Moreover the red cells can be resuspended into a solution designed to offer optimal conditions for red cell storage, e.g. saline-adenine-glucose-mannitol (SAGM). The resuspension may still be done within the closed system. Cell-free plasma can now be frozen and be stored as fresh frozen plasma to be used as such or as a starting material for further products.

Table 3(b) provides an estimation of the results that can be obtained using initial centrifugation (4 options) or filtration (1 option).

Depending on the choice of technique for component preparation:

- methods I and II will be followed by recentrifugation of the platelet-rich plasma for the preparation of cell-free plasma and platelet concentrate;

- method III will be followed by preparation of platelet concentrate from buffy coats.

5.2   *Separation after initial filtration*

Whole blood may be filtered for leukocyte depletion prior to high speed centrifugation. This procedure enables a separation into almost cell-free plasma and leukocyte-depleted (and platelet depleted) red cells.

<u>Table 3(b):</u> Five different methods of initial separation of whole blood and the approximate composition of the fractions obtained (figures refer to a standard donation of 450 ml ± 10% taken into 60-70 ml of anticoagulant).

Method	I	II	III	IV	V
Initial Filtration	no	no	no	no	yes
Centrifugation speed	low	low	high	high	high
Separation into	plasma + buffy coat + red cells	plasma + red cells	plasma + buffy coat + red cells	plasma + red cells	plasma + red cells leukocyte depleted
Resulting crude fractions:					
- plasma, volume	200-280 ml	200-280 ml	270-320 ml	270-330 ml	240-290 ml
- platelets	70-80%	70-80%	10-20%	10-20%	<1%
- leukocytes	5-10%	5-10%	2-5%	2-5%	<0.01%
Red cells:					
- Hct*	0.75-0.80	0.65-0.75	0.85-0.90	0.80-0.90	0.80-0.90
- platelets	5-15%	20-30%	10-20%	80-90%	<1%
- leukocytes	25-45%	90-95%	25-45%	95-98%	<0.01%
Buffy coat:					
- Hct*	50-70%		40-60%		
- red cells	10-15%		10-15%		
- platelets	10-25%		80-90%		
- leukocytes	60-70%		50-70%		

*   Haematocrit

5.3 Other separation principles

Zonal centrifugation

Sedimentation of blood cells can be achieved when a centrifugal force is exerted on flowing blood more or less perpendicular to the direction of the flow. The efficiency of the separation depends on the ratio between the centrifugal force and the flow velocity. At a high ratio the plasma obtained is platelet poor, and at a lower ratio platelet rich plasma can be obtained.

A number of apheresis devices are available in which this principle is applied for the production of cell poor plasma or platelet rich plasma.

A further application of zonal centrifugation is the removal of plasma protein from a blood cell suspension. A unit of blood cells is introduced into the centrifuge bowl; a flow of washing fluid is then maintained until the protein concentration in the effluent is sufficiently reduced. Centrifugation is discontinued and the "washed" blood cell suspension is harvested.

The same principle is also used for both the addition and the removal of cryoprotectant before freezing and after thawing of blood cell suspensions in cryopreservation.

Buoyant density centrifugation

Buoyant density centrifugation of blood, bone marrow or buffy coat cells on top of a layer with a density of 1.077 g/ml leads to a layer of mononuclear cells floating on the interface and a pellet of red cells and granulocytes which have penetrated through the separating medium according to the density of the cells involved.

Buoyant density separation is generally applicable for separations based on density differences between cells e.g. also for the separation of cells complexed with red cells to rosettes from the non-rosetted cells.

Counter current centrifugation (elutriation)

Cells, subjected simultaneously to a liquid flow and a centrifugal force in opposite directions, tend to be separated according to their size. This property has been applied in cell separators to collect apheresis platelet concentrates with a reduced leukocyte content, which, for some devices, may reach the specification of leukocyte depletion, i.e. $<10^6$ leukocytes/unit.

Using specific centrifuges, counter current centrifugation is also used to separate subpopulations of mononuclear cells obtained from blood or bone marrow.

Filtration

At present, two major types of filtration are available for blood component preparation:

- the separation of plasma from blood by cross-flow filtration;
- the removal of leukocytes from cell suspensions by depth-filtration or surface filtration.

Cross-flow filtration

When blood flows along a membrane with a pore size allowing free passage of plasma proteins but not of blood cells, cell-free plasma may be obtained by filtration.

Plasmapheresis devices have been developed in which a pumping system takes blood from the donor's vein, mixes it at a constant ratio with anti-coagulant solution and then leads it along a plasma-permeable membrane (flat membrane or hollow fibre system). Two pressures are exerted on the blood: one parallel to the membrane, keeping the blood flowing along the membrane, and the other perpendicular to the membrane, the actual filtration pressure. This system prevents accumulation of cells on the membrane while plasma is removed from the blood (the haematocrit in the system may increase from 0.40 to 0.75). In some devices, velocity of the flow parallel to the membrane is increased by an additional vortex action or by movement of the membrane.

When a specified extra-corporeal cell volume has been reached, the cells are reinfused to the donor, and the next cycle starts until the required volume of cell-free plasma has been obtained.

Depth and surface filtration

Owing to the specific properties of platelets and granulocytes as well as the low flexibility of lymphocytes, these cells are more easily trapped in a filter bed of fibres than red cells. Four mechanisms of trapping have been recognised in filters used for leukocyte depletion of red cell concentrates:

a)   the activation of platelets leading to the attachment of these cells to the fibres in the top of the filter, followed by the interaction of the attached platelets and granulocytes;

b)   the activation of granulocytes by another type of fibre leading to attachment of these cells in the middle part of the filter;

c)   the obstruction of the lymphocytes in the pores and fork junctions of the finest fibre material in the bottom layers of the filter. Blow-moulded mats of fibre material with different pore sizes and fibre thicknesses are now used to produce leukocyte depletion filters for red cell concentrates;

d)   surface treatment of the filter material allows the production of filters which reduce the contaminating leukocytes from platelet concentrates by sieving and may prevent activation of platelets.

Filters used for leukocyte removal from red cells or platelets show considerable variations in efficacy and capacity. Besides filter properties, the final result of filtration is influenced by several process parameters (e.g., flow rate, temperature, priming and rinsing) and properties of the component to be filtered (e.g. storage history of the component, number of leukocytes and number of platelets). When a standardised filtration procedure is established, limits must therefore be set for all the variables affecting the efficacy of filtration and the Standard Operating Procedures (SOPs) should be fully validated under the condition to be used.

Leukocyte depleted components

The introduction of any leukocyte depletion process either by filtration or special centrifugation technique needs careful validation. An appropriate method should be used for leukocyte counting after leukocyte depletion. This method should be validated.

The validation should be carried out by the blood establishment using the manufacturer's instructions against the requirements for leukocyte depletion and other quality aspects of the components including plasma for fractionation.

To enable comparison of filters aimed at leukocyte depletion and to allow selection between them, the manufacturers should report data on their system performance under defined conditions. Manufacturers should also provide performance data to the blood establishment on variations between different modifications to a given filter type and between batches.

Mathematical models have been developed to calculate the sample size necessary to validate and control the leukocyte depletion process.

After full validation of the process, tools such as statistical process control could be used in ongoing process control to detect any change in the process and/or the procedures.

Particular problems may arise with donations from donors with red cell abnormalities (e.g. sickle-cell trait) where adequate leukocyte depletion may not be achieved and more detailed quality control procedures are necessary (e.g. leukocyte counting of every donation). The quality of the red cells following filtration processes needs further investigation.

Washing of cellular components

This technique is occasionally used when there is requirement for cellular blood components with a very low level of plasma protein.

6.   Cryoprecipitation

The isolation of some plasma proteins, most importantly Factor VIII, fibronectin and fibrinogen, can be achieved by making use of their reduced solubility at low temperature. In practice, this is done by freezing units of plasma, thawing and centrifugation at low temperature.

Details regarding the freezing, thawing, and centrifugation conditions required for cryoprecipitate production, are provided under Chapter 16: Cryoprecipitate.

7.   Freezing and thawing of plasma

7.1   Rationale

Freezing is a critical step in the conservation of plasma Factor VIII. During freezing, pure ice is formed and the plasma solutes are concentrated in the remaining water. When the solubility of the solutes is exceeded, each solute forms crystals but may be influenced by the used anticoagulants. Further studies on this aspect are ongoing.

The ice formation depends on the rate of heat extraction, whereas the diffusion rates of the solutes determine their displacement. At slow freezing rates, the diffusion of solutes copes with the rate of ice formation; solutes are increasingly concentrated in the middle of a plasma unit.

Since all solutes are displaced simultaneously, the Factor VIII molecules are exposed to a high concentration of salts for a prolonged time and thus inactivated. At a high freezing rate, the ice formation overtakes the solute displacement and small clusters of solidified solute are homogeneously trapped in the ice without prolonged contact between highly concentrated salts and Factor VIII.

To achieve the highest yield of Factor VIII, plasma should be frozen to -30°C or below.

Decrease of Factor VIII during freezing occurs when the solidification of plasma takes more than one hour. This can be monitored by measuring the total protein content of a core sample of the frozen plasma; this protein concentration should be identical with the total protein content of plasma before freezing. An optimal freezing rate is obtainable when a heat extraction of 38 kcal per hour per unit of plasma is achieved, and can be monitored by the use of thermocouples.

In order to effectively incorporate these techniques into a coherent daily routine, the blood bank staff has to be familiar with the thinking behind the technique as well as its potential limitations and pitfalls.

7.2   Methods of freezing

When freezing plasma, the rate of cooling should be as rapid as possible and optimally should bring the core temperature down to -30°C or below within 60 minutes.

Experience has shown that without the use of a snap-freezer it takes several hours to reach this temperature. The time can be reduced, for example by the following means:

- plasma should be presented in a regular configuration to maximise exposure to the freezing process (e.g. bags laid flat or in formers if vertical);

- immersion in an environment at very low temperature;

- if a liquid environment is used, it should have been shown that the container cannot be penetrated by the solvent.

As for the required storage conditions, reference is made to Chapter 3, 14.3 and the individual monographs.

7.3   Methods of thawing

Frozen units should be handled with care since the bags may be brittle. The integrity of the pack should be verified before and after thawing to exclude any defects and leakages. Containers which leak must be discarded. The product should be thawed immediately after removal from storage in a properly controlled environment at +37°C according to a validated procedure. After thawing of frozen plasma, the content should be inspected to ensure that no insoluble cryoprecipitate is visible on completion of the thaw procedure.

The product should not be used if insoluble material is present. In order to preserve labile factors, plasma should be used immediately following thawing and never beyond 6 hours. It should not be refrozen.

Thawing of the plasma is an inevitable part of some of the current viral inactivation processes. The final component, having been refrozen after treatment, should be used immediately following thawing for clinical use and not further refrozen.

8.   The use of an open system and devices for sterile connections

It is suggested that any new development in component preparation involving an open system should be subjected to intensive testing during the developmental phase for maintenance of sterility.

Blood components prepared by an open system should be used as quickly as possible.

Components prepared in systems using fully validated sterile connecting devices may be stored as if prepared in a closed system. Monitoring should be carried out by pressure testing of all connections and regular traction tests.

9.   Other methods

9.1   *Gamma-irradiated blood components - prevention of GVHD*

Viable lymphocytes in blood products can cause fatal graft-versus-host reaction in severely immuno-compromised patients, e.g. patients receiving immunosuppressive therapy, children with severe immuno-deficiency syndromes and low birth-weight neonates. Other categories of patients are also at risk of this rare complication e.g. following intrauterine transfusion, transfusion between family members and transfusion of HLA- matched components.

Lymphocytes can be rendered non-viable by exposure to ionising radiation. This treatment does not cause significant harm to other blood components and an irradiated component can therefore safely be given to all patients.

The protocol should ensure that no part of the component receives a dose less than 25 Gray or more than 50 Gray. Exposure time must be standardised for each radiation source and re-validated at suitable intervals to take decay of the isotope into account.

Red cell products may be irradiated up to 14 days after collection and thereafter stored until the 28th day after collection. In view of the increased potassium leak from red cells consequent to their irradiation, such cells intended for intrauterine or massive neonatal transfusion should be used within 48 hours of irradiation.

Irradiated platelets can be used up to their original expiry date.

The use of radiation-sensitive labels to demonstrate that the component has been irradiated is recommended.

9.2   Cytomegalovirus-free blood components

Cytomegalovirus (CMV) is a common infectious agent that can be transmitted by transfusion of blood components. The risk of disease transmission is highest with fresh products containing mono- and polynuclear leukocytes. CMV infection is often asymptomatic in healthy persons. Antibodies usually appear 4 to 8 weeks after infection and can be demonstrated in standard screening tests. Since the infection is common, the test has to be repeated on each donation from a previously sero-negative donor.

Infection caused by this virus is usually not clinically significant in immuno-competent recipients, but can cause severe, even fatal, disease in certain patients not previously exposed to the virus:

- transplant recipients;
- patients with severe immuno-deficiency;
- foetus (intra-uterine transfusion);
- anti-CMV negative pregnant women;
- low weight premature infants and neonates.

These patients should receive components selected or processed to minimise risk of CMV infectivity. Use of components from anti-CMV negative donors or leukocyte depleted products significantly reduces the risk of CMV-transmission and CMV-disease in immunocompromised patients. However, neither method nor the combination can completely avoid transmission from occasional case of CMV-viremia in the early stage of acute infection.

9.3   Pathogen reduction

Systems exist that will reduce or inactivate a wide range of microbial pathogens in blood components. However, it is recognised that the relative benefits and risks of pathogen reduction procedures are not fully established. These procedures are not currently available for all blood components. National transfusion services should decide individually about the value for implementation of these systems in the given context.

10.   Definitions and minimum requirements

Since blood components are used to correct a known deficit, each preparation must be subjected to strict quality control. The aim is to produce "pure" components, but a very high degree of purity can be difficult and expensive to obtain and might not even be necessary in all instances. However, it is absolutely necessary to declare the quality and to be able to make different types of preparations in order to give the clinicians a reasonable choice for patients with different transfusion demands.

For example, a red cell concentrate can be produced with varying concentrations of contaminating leukocytes and platelets. A buffy coat depleted preparation where the majority of the leukocytes and the platelets have been removed is useful to the majority of recipients since microaggregate formation during storage will be inhibited. If the patient has antibodies against leukocyte antigens or if it can be foreseen that he/she will need a very large number of transfusions, leukocyte depletion must be much more efficient.

In order to institute an adequate scheme of component therapy, all products must be carefully defined and minimum requirements set. Clinical users should be informed of the properties of all components.

11.   Introducing component preparation in a blood bank

Laboratories with little or no experience of component preparation should allow their staff to attend training courses and visit blood banks with extensive experience of work of this type.

Equipment should be purchased with provision for adequate service and maintenance. A method must be chosen which will achieve the desired results. All steps in the procedure should be clearly explained in a manual which should be available at the work bench.

Before the method is taken into routine use, it must be fully validated and a Standard Operating Procedure (SOP) established. Each prepared unit must be carefully checked until it is verified that the intended quality is obtained. Routinely prepared products should then be subjected to regular quality control.

12.   Product control - quality assurance

In all respects the preparation of blood products and components should follow the principles of Good Manufacturing Practice (GMP) including implementation of Statistical Process Control (SPC) as defined in Chapter 27.

The purpose of product control is to help the blood bank maintain a high and even quality of the prepared product. In this way, clinical outcome will improve, confidence in component therapy will increase and the introduction of an adequate component therapy programme will be facilitated.

Lack of accuracy, deviation from SOP or incorrect handling when blood is processed will not give the intended component quality.

Method descriptions and product control go hand in hand; therefore an SOP for product control is also necessary. The results of product control must be continuously evaluated and steps taken to correct defective procedures or equipment.

Care should be taken of using fully standardised laboratory techniques for the quality assessment of blood components. The suitability of each method to provide the intended information must be validated.

In the following chapters, the different blood components will be defined and described. Principles of good preparation methods, storage and transport will also be described, and finally guidelines for quality control will be given.

13. Microbiological safety of blood components

Although blood collection and processing procedures are intended to produce non-infectious blood components, bacterial contamination still may occur. Bacterial quality control testing in all blood components may be appropriate. However, for whole blood collection, bacterial cultures of platelets provide the best indication of the overall rate of contamination, provided that the sample for culture is obtained on a suitable sample volume and at a suitable time post-collection. Surveillance studies have found rates of contamination as high as 0.4% in single donor platelets, although rates at or below 0.2% more often have been reported. The causes include occult bacteraemia in the donor, inadequate or contaminated skin preparation at the phlebotomy site, coring of a skin plug by the phlebotomy needle, and breaches of the closed system from equipment defects or mishandling. Platelet products are more likely than other blood components to be associated with sepsis due to their storage at room temperature, which is permissive of bacterial growth.

A variety of procedures may be used to obtain a valid platelet sample for bacterial culture. Aseptic techniques are required in order to minimise the risk of false positive cultures due to contamination at the time of sampling or upon inoculation in culture. Additionally, it is prudent to retain a sample that can be used for repeat culture to validate a positive result. Large volume samples removed from a several unit platelet pool or single donor apheresis unit can be cultured any time post collection. However small volume samples (e.g. 2-5 ml removed from a single whole blood unit) should be taken for culture after a 48 hour delay post-collection. The delayed sampling of a small volume permits bacterial growth to a level that subsequent assays will reliably detect, thereby overcoming sampling errors at low contamination levels.

13.1 Quality control for Aseptic Collection and Processing of Blood Components

The goal of quality control testing for bacterial contamination should be to assure that blood collection and processing procedures conform to current standards. Statistically defined sampling of platelets for culture (or nucleic acid testing) by a validated method will provide a reliable indication of the rate of contamination for all the blood components. Quality control testing may be of value in long term process control, if validated and conducted according to an appropriate statistical plan.

Based on these considerations one possible approach for monitoring this issue is as follows:

a) *As a quality control for aseptic collection of blood components, blood collection centres should determine the rate of bacterial contamination in platelets at least yearly by culturing 1,500 or more units (about 30 units per week or 5% of units released after 48 hours of storage, whichever is larger.) Standard statistical methods should be used to identify significant deviations from a baseline contamination rate not to exceed 0.2%. The chosen method should be based on a predetermined level of confidence to exclude a maximum tolerated rate of contamination, and an action limit should be established.*

b) *All instances of a positive culture should be investigated promptly to identify a correctable cause.*

c) *Whenever the observed rate of bacterial contamination exceeds the defined action limit, a comprehensive investigation into potential causes of contamination should be undertaken and all collection and processing procedures should be revalidated.*

Example:

A blood centre wishes to establish surveillance to detect bacterial contamination rates significantly in excess of 0.2%. The following chart is derived from binomial statistics:

Candidate Action Limit #(+)/# sampled	Confidence in Positive Result	Power to detect actual contamination rate @			
		0.4%	0.6%	0.8%	1.0%
≥3 per 400	95.3%	22%	43%	62%	76%
≥5 per 800	97.6%	22%	52%	77%	90%
≥7 per 1600	95.5%	46%	84%	97%	99.6%

The blood centre collects 12 units of platelets per day, five days per week. Cultures of units released after 48 hours, plus outdated units, number 30 units per week that are processed as 6 weekly cultures of five unit pools. An action limit is set to revalidate the collection procedures if the observed contamination rate exceeds 0.42% for yearly samples of 1,560 units. The action limit was established based on an expected contamination rate of 0.2%, a sample size of 1,560, and a cut-off determined as baseline plus 2-sigma variation. For this scheme, the likelihood of rejecting a conforming process is 4.5% (once every 22 years). The confidence levels (i.e. power) to exclude actual contamination rates of 1%, 0.8% and 0.6% are 99.6%, 97% and 84% respectively.

Over a one-year period, 7 positive platelet pools are identified, traceable to 7 individual units. The individual cases were investigated, but no attributable cause was identified. The observed contamination rate of 7/1,560=0.45% exceeds the action level. Confidence that the actual contamination rate exceeds 0.2% is greater than 95%. An intensive review is conducted, and all collection and processing procedures are revalidated.

13.2   *"Culture-Negative to Date" - "Release"*

Routine pre-release bacteriological testing of all platelets to establish a criterion for issue of platelets as "culture-negative to date" obviates recommendations a, b, and c in section 13.1. Sampling of platelets for the purpose of establishing a release criterion based on a negative result of bacterial cultures requires that the integrity of the closed system should be maintained. This is because platelets may continue to be stored for a variable period after sampling and before use. Suitable methods of sampling in this case would include the use of integral satellite containers, or stripping, refilling, and then pinching off duplicate pigtails. Sampling also may be done into collection containers via the use of sterile connecting devices consistent with Chapter 3, paragraph 8.

14.   Storage of blood components

Storage conditions for blood components must be designed to preserve optimal viability and function during the whole storage period. The risk of bacterial contamination decreases substantially if only closed separation and storage systems are used. Storage routines must also be controlled continuously, as should issue and return routines; transport of blood components must also take place in a safe and controlled way.

14.1   *Equipment*

Blood components are stored at +20°C to +24°C, at +2°C to +6°C or at different temperatures below 0°C. Whatever type of storage device is chosen, the following points should be considered before purchase:

i.   refrigerators and freezers must have surplus capacity. The space should be easy to inspect;

ii.   the operation must be reliable and temperature distribution must be uniform within the unit;

iii.   the equipment must have temperature recording and alarm devices;

iv.   the equipment should be easy to clean and should withstand strong detergents. It should also conform to local safety requirements.

14.2   Storage at +2 °C to +6 °C

Refrigerators for blood component storage should be restricted to whole blood, blood components, and sample tubes. Test reagents and kits should be stored in separate refrigeration units.

Separate space should be reserved for:

- units for issue;
- units selected for certain patients including autologous donations;
- units kept in quarantine awaiting completion of testing;
- outdated and discarded units.

The space for each of these component types should be clearly indicated. The temperature within the unit should be recorded continuously. The sensor of the thermograph should be placed within a blood bag filled with 10% glycerol solution to a volume of 250 ml or a volume equivalent to the normal volume of the stored component. This container should be placed in the upper part of the refrigerated space. In large refrigerated rooms, two such sensors should be applied.

The alarm system should preferably have both acoustic and optical signals and should be tested regularly.

Refrigerators for blood components should ideally be connected to a reserve power unit as well as the main supply.

14.3   Storage of frozen plasma components

The eutectic point of plasma is -23°C. To allow for temperature fluctuation during use, a transfusion centre should have a freezer routinely capable of running at below -30°C.

The freezers should not contain non-therapeutic products. Separate space should be allocated for the different types of products and be clearly marked to avoid mistakes.

Freezers with automatic defrosting should be avoided unless it can be guaranteed that the low temperature is maintained during defrosting.

The temperature within the freezer should be recorded continuously. The alarm system should preferably have both acoustic and optical signals, and should be tested regularly.

Freezers should ideally be connected to a reserve power source as well as the main supply.

14.4   Storage at +20°C to +24°C

Platelets are stored at +20°C to +24°C. A closed device that permits temperature control is recommended. If such a device is unavailable, the space chosen should be capable of maintaining the required constant temperature.

The platelets should be stored in agitators which should:

- enable satisfactory mixing in the bag as well as gas exchange through the wall of the bag;

- avoid folding of the bags;

- have a set speed to avoid foaming.

A closed device should have thermograph and alarm systems. Otherwise, a control thermometer should be used at the storage site and checked several times daily. The speed of the agitator should be tested regularly according to the manufacturer's recommendations and failure should be monitored.

14.5   Aspects of red cell preservation

The anticoagulant solutions used in blood collection have been developed to prevent coagulation and to permit storage of red cells for a certain period of time. While originally designed for whole blood storage, they have also been used in blood from which components are prepared. All of the solutions contain sodium citrate, citric acid and glucose, some of them may also contain adenine, guanosine and phosphate.

Citrate binds calcium and prevents clotting of the blood. Glucose is used by the red cell during storage and each glucose molecule gives two molecules of adenosine tri-phosphate (ATP) which is formed by phosphorylation of adenosine di-phosphate (ADP). ATP is an energy-rich molecule which is used to support the energy-demanding functions of the erythrocyte, such as membrane flexibility and certain membrane transport functions. During its action in energy-consuming operations, ATP is transferred back to ADP. Citric acid is added to the anticoagulant in order to obtain a hydrogen ion concentration which is suitably high at the beginning of storage at +4°C.

Without this addition the blood would be too alkaline at storage temperature.

During storage, an increasing acidity occurs which reduces glycolysis. The content of adenosine nucleotides (ATP, ADP, AMP) decreases during storage. By addition of adenine which is a main component in the adenosine nucleotides, the erythrocytes can synthesise new AMP, ADP and ATP and compensate for (or reduce) the losses.

When red cell concentrates are prepared, a considerable part of the glucose and adenine is removed with the plasma. If not compensated for in other ways (e.g. larger amount than normal of adenine and glucose in the anticoagulant or by separate addition of a suspension/preservative medium), sufficient viability of the red cells can only be maintained if the cells are not over-concentrated. Normal CPD-adenine red cell concentrate should therefore not have an Hct above 0.70 on average. This also keeps the viscosity sufficiently low to permit transfusion of the concentrate without pre-administration dilution.

Platelets and leukocytes rapidly lose their viability at +4°C. They form microaggregates which are present in considerable amounts even after 3 to 4 days' storage of whole blood and even more so in red cell concentrates. Microaggregates can pass through the filters of ordinary blood transfusion sets. They are considered to be able to cause decreased lung function by blocking the lung capillaries and this may be of clinical importance in massive transfusions. Removal of platelets during component preparation reduces microaggregate formation. Likewise, leukocyte depletion by buffy coat removal will also reduce the frequency of febrile transfusion reactions and will help in obtaining high-grade depletion of leukocytes when leukocyte-removal filters are used for this purpose.

An additive or suspension medium allows maintenance of red cell viability even if more than 90% of the plasma is removed. The use of glucose and adenine is necessary for the maintenance of red blood cell post-transfusion viability, phosphate may be used to enhance glycolysis, and other substances may be used to prevent in vitro haemolysis (i.e. mannitol, citrate). Sodium chloride or di-sodium phosphate may be used to give the additive solution a suitable osmotic strength.

14.6 Erythrocyte preparations

Red cells may be stored in the fluid state at a controlled temperature of +2°C to +6°C. The performance of the storage refrigerator must itself be carefully controlled (see Chapter 24). The maximum duration of storage (expiry date) should be noted on each container. This duration may vary with the type of preparation (concentration of cells, formula of anticoagulant, use of additive suspension fluid, etc.) and should be determined for each type on the basis of achieving a mean 24 hours post-transfusion survival of no less than 75% of the transfused red cells.

Red cells in the frozen state should be prepared and reconstituted according to an approved protocol, be stored at -80°C or below, and produce satisfactory post-transfusion survival figures.

14.7   Platelet preparations

Platelet preparations are particularly sensitive to storage conditions. Platelet metabolism, and consequently post-transfusion function and viability, is dependent on adequate oxygen availability, the temperature and the pH of the platelet preparation.

When stored at +22°C, 100×10^9 platelets consume approximately 10 μmoles of oxygen per hour. The platelet demand for oxygen may be influenced by different agitation modes and varying pH and temperature. Addition of acetate to the storage medium may increase the oxygen consumption. Contaminating leukocytes also consume oxygen but the small number present in a platelet storage bag contributes little to the total need for oxygen.

When the number of platelets in a storage bag exceeds the number that can safely be supplied with oxygen, the glucose consumption increases three to five times, resulting in a rapid lactic acid production, decreasing pH, fall in ATP concentration and loss of platelet viability.

Thus, the maximum number of platelets to be stored is limited by the oxygen diffusion capacity of the platelet storage bag. When a new plastic bag is introduced for platelet preservation, the maximum number of platelets that may be stored in that bag should be determined for different modes of preparation and agitation, suspension media and pH.

The use of special gas-permeable plastic containers, proper temperature (+20°C to +24°C) and adequate agitation during storage are all features necessary for proper storage of this component.

14.8   Granulocyte preparations

Ordinarily, granulocyte suspensions are prepared for a specific patient and administered immediately. If intermediate storage is unavoidable this should be at a controlled +20°C to +24°C for a maximum of 24 hours. Granulocytes should not be agitated on a platelet rocker.

14.9   Plasma components

Recommended storage conditions for fresh frozen plasma and cryoprecipitate and for cryoprecipitate-depleted plasma are given in Table 3(c).

<u>Table 3(c)</u>:   *Recommended storage conditions*

Product	Length of storage and temperature
Fresh frozen plasma, cryoprecipitate and cryoprecipitate-depleted plasma	36 months at below -25 °C

3 months at -18 °C to -25 °C |

<u>Note</u>:   The recommended temperature ranges are based upon practical refrigeration conditions. Ideally the surface temperature of the product should not rise above the eutectic point of -23 °C (e.g. during opening of freezers, etc.).

Validations on the exact relation between storage times and temperature are pending.

For plasma intended for fractionation refer to the appropriate European Pharmacopoeia monograph.

15.   Issue and transportation

Blood components should be transported by a system which has been validated to maintain the recommended storage temperature of the component over the proposed maximum time and extremes of ambient temperature of transport. The containers used in transport should be well insulated, easy to clean and easy to handle. Where a dedicated refrigerated vehicle is used the principles applying to control of the refrigerators should be observed. Alternatively, systems for road or rail transport using controlled cooling elements may be considered. These coolants must not come into close contact with the blood bags.

Red cell components should be kept between +2°C and +6°C. Validated transport systems should ensure that at the end of a maximum transit time of 24 hours the temperature should not have exceeded +10°C. Platelet components should be kept between +20°C and +24°C and frozen plasma transported in the frozen state as close as possible to the recommended storage temperature (see appropriate chapters).

Transport conditions and containers should be validated. It is recommended that some form of temperature indicator be used to monitor the in-transit temperature. On receipt, if not intended for immediate transfusion, the product should be transferred to storage under recommended conditions.

The temperature on receipt can be monitored as follows:

- Take 2 bags from the container, place a thermometer between the bags and fix them together with rubber bands. Quickly replace them into the container and close the lid. Read the temperature after 5 minutes. The temperature of red cell bags should not go below +1°C nor exceed +10°C. Alternatively an electronic sensing device may be used to take immediate measurements from the surface of a pack.

Returned blood components should not be reissued for transfusion if the bag has been penetrated or entered, the product not maintained continuously within the approved temperature range or if there is evidence of leakage, abnormal colour change or excess haemolysis. The proper identification, time of issue and transit history should be fully documented.

16. Component information and principles of labelling

Brief information about the various blood components should be made available to clinicians with regard to composition, indications, storage and transfusion practices.

This would include that the blood must not be used for transfusion if there is abnormal haemolysis or other deterioration and that all blood components must be administered through a 170-200 μm filter, if not otherwise stated. The information should be presented to the clinicians in a booklet and/or in a product information leaflet.

The labelling of blood components should comply with the relevant national legislation and international agreements. Each single blood container must be uniquely identified by the identity number and the component description, preferably in eye and machine readable codes, allowing full traceability to the donor and the collection, testing, processing, storage, release, distribution and transfusion of the blood component.

The label on the component ready for distribution should contain eye readable information necessary for safe transfusion, i.e. the unique identity number (preferably consisting of a code for the responsible blood collection organisation, the year of donation and a serial number), the ABO and RhD blood group, the name of the blood component and essential information about the properties and handling of the blood component, the expiry date.

PART C:
Blood components

Chapter 4: Whole blood

Definition

Whole blood for transfusion is blood taken from a suitable donor using a sterile and pyrogen-free anticoagulant and container. The major use of whole blood is as source material for blood component preparation.

Properties

Freshly drawn whole blood maintains all its properties for a limited period of time. Rapid deterioration of Factor VIII, leukocytes and platelets makes whole blood an unsuitable product for treatment of haemostatic disturbances when stored beyond the first 24 hours. Upon further liquid storage a number of changes occur, such as increase of oxygen affinity and loss of viability of the red cells, loss of coagulation factor activity (Factors VIII and V), loss of platelet viability and function, formation of microaggregates, release of intracellular components such as potassium and leukocyte proteases, and activation of plasma factors such as kallikrein.

Whole blood for transfusion should not contain irregular antibodies of clinical significance.

Methods of preparation

Whole blood for transfusion is used without further processing.

Labelling

The labelling should comply with the relevant national legislation and international agreements. The following information should be shown on the label or contained in the product information leaflet, as appropriate:

- the producer's identification;
- the unique identity number;
- the ABO and RhD group;
- the date of donation;
- the name of the anticoagulant solution;
- the name of the blood component;
- additional component information: irradiated, etc. (if appropriate);
- the date of expiry;

- the volume or weight of the blood component;

- the temperature of storage;

- blood group phenotypes other than ABO and RhD (optional);

- that the component must not be used for transfusion if there is abnormal haemolysis or other deterioration;

- that the component must be administered through a 170-200 μm filter.

Storage and stability

During storage, the temperature of the blood component should remain between +2°C to +6°C. The storage time depends on the anticoagulant/preservative solution used. For CPD-A 1 the storage time is 35 days.

Microaggregates are formed on storage.

During storage there is a progressive decrease in the labile coagulation factors V and VIII, an increase in potassium and acidity in the plasma and a rapid decrease in platelet viability because of storage at +2°C to +6°C.

The haemoglobin oxygen release function is impaired during storage due to progressive loss of 2,3-bisphosphoglycerate (2,3-BPG, previous name 2,3-diphosphoglycerate, DPG). After 10 days of storage in CPD-A 1 all 2,3 BPG is lost. However, it regenerates after transfusion in the circulation of the recipient.

Quality control

Much of the quality control necessary to ensure the safety and efficacy of whole blood takes place at the time of blood collection. In addition to the measures carried out at the time of collection, the parameters listed in Table 4 must also be checked.

Table 4:

Parameter to be checked	Quality requirement	Frequency of control	Control executed by
ABO, RhD	Grouping	All units	grouping lab
anti-HIV 1&2	Negative by approved screening test	All units	screening lab
HBsAg	Negative by approved screening test	All units	screening lab
anti-HBc (when required)	Negative by approved screening test	All units	screening lab
anti-HCV	Negative by approved screening test	All units	screening lab
Syphilis (when required)	Negative by screening test	All units	screening lab
anti-CMV (when required)	Negative by screening test	As required	screening lab
anti-HTLV I&II (when required)	Negative by screening test	All units	screening lab
Volume	450 ml ± 10% volume excluding anticoagulant A non-standard donation should be labelled accordingly	1% of all units with a minimum of 4 units per month	processing lab
Haemoglobin	Minimum 45 g/unit	4 units per month	QC lab
Haemolysis at the end of storage	<0.8% of red cell mass	4 units per month	QC lab

Transport

After collection, blood should be kept at a controlled temperature, between +2°C and +6°C. Validated transport systems should ensure that at the end of a maximum transit time of 24 hours the temperature should not have exceeded +10°C. Alternatively, whole blood can be kept up to 24 hours in conditions validated to maintain temperature between +20°C and +24°C, a prerequisite for the production of platelet preparations from whole blood.

Indications for use

Where component preparation is routine, whole blood must be considered as a source material and has no, or only a very restricted, place in transfusion practice. In the absence of appropriate plasma substitutes and blood components, the use of whole blood can only be envisaged in clinical settings where red cell and blood volume deficit are simultaneously present.

Precautions in use

Compatibility of whole blood with the intended recipient must be verified by suitable pre-transfusion testing.

Whole blood is contra-indicated in:

- anaemia without blood volume loss;
- various types of plasma intolerance;
- intolerance due to alloimmunisation against leukocyte antigens.

Side-effects

- circulatory overload;
- haemolytic transfusion reactions;
- non-haemolytic transfusion reaction (mainly chills, fever and urticaria);
- sepsis by inadvertent bacterial contamination of blood;
- syphilis can be transmitted when whole blood has been stored for less than 96 hours at +4°C;
- viral transmission (hepatitis, HIV, etc.) is possible despite careful donor selection and screening procedures;
- protozoal transmission (e.g. malaria) may occur in rare instances;
- alloimmunisation against HLA and red cell antigens;
- citrate intoxication in neonates and in patients with impaired liver function;
- biochemical imbalance in massive transfusion, e.g. hyperkalaemia;
- post-transfusion purpura;
- T.R.A.L.I. (Transfusion Related Acute Lung Injury);
- transmission of other pathogens that are not tested for or recognised.

Chapter 5: Red cells

Definition

A component obtained by removal of part of the plasma from whole blood, without further processing.

Properties

The haematocrit (Hct) of the component is 0.65-0.75. Each unit should have a minimum of 45 g of haemoglobin at the end of processing.

The unit contains all of the original unit's red cells. The greater part of its leukocytes (about 2.5 to 3.0 × 10^9 cells) and a varying content of platelets depending on the method of centrifugation are retained, no effort having been made for removal.

Methods of preparation

For the preparation of the component, removal of the plasma from the whole blood unit after centrifugation is performed. Whole blood can be kept up to 24 hours in conditions validated to maintain a temperature between + 20°C to + 24°C.

Labelling

The labelling should comply with the relevant national legislation and international agreements. The following information should be shown on the label or contained in the product information leaflet, as appropriate:

- the producer's identification;
- the unique identity number;
- the ABO and RhD group;
- the date of donation;
- the name of the anticoagulant solution;
- the name of the blood component;
- additional component information: irradiated, etc. (if appropriate);
- the date of expiry;
- the volume or weight of the blood component;
- the temperature of storage;

- blood group phenotypes other than ABO and RhD (optional);
- that the component must not be used for transfusion if there is abnormal haemolysis or other deterioration;
- that the component must be administered through a 170-200 μm filter.

Storage and stability

As for whole blood. Microaggregates are formed on storage.

Quality control

As for whole blood with the exceptions indicated in Table 5.

Table 5:

Parameter to be checked	Quality requirement (specification)	Frequency of control	Control executed by
Volume	280 ± 50 ml	1% of all units	Processing lab
Hct	0.65 to 0.75	4 units per month	QC lab
Haemoglobin	minimum 45 g/unit	4 units per month	QC lab
Haemolysis at the end of storage	<0.8% of red cell mass	4 units per month	QC lab

Transport

For red cells that have been stored in a refrigerated container, validated transport systems should ensure that at the end of a maximum transit time of 24 hours the temperature should not have exceeded +10°C.

Transport by a non-refrigerated vehicle requires a cooled and insulated container.

Indications for use

Red cells are used for replacement in blood loss and for the therapy of anaemia.

Precautions in use

Compatibility of red cells with the intended recipient must be verified by suitable pre-transfusion testing.

Red cells are not recommended in:

- various types of plasma intolerance;
- intolerance due to alloimmunisation against leukocyte antigens;
- exchange transfusion in newborns unless supplementary plasma is added.

Side-effects

- circulatory overload;
- haemolytic transfusion reaction;
- non-haemolytic transfusion reaction (mainly chills, fever);
- alloimmunisation against HLA and red cell antigens;
- syphilis can be transmitted when red cells have been stored for less than 96 hours at +4°C;
- viral transmission (hepatitis, HIV, etc.) is possible despite careful donor selection and screening procedures;
- protozoal transmission (e.g. malaria) may occur in rare instances;
- sepsis due to inadvertent bacterial contamination;
- biochemical imbalance in massive transfusion, e.g. hyperkalaemia;
- post-transfusion purpura;
- T.R.A.L.I. (Transfusion Related Acute Lung Injury);
- transmission of other pathogens that are not tested for or recognised.

Chapter 6: Red cells, buffy coat removed

Definition

A component prepared by the separation of part of the plasma and the buffy-coat layer from red cells.

Properties

The Hct of the component is 0.65 to 0.75.

The unit contains all, except 10 to 30 ml, of the original unit's red cells. Each unit should have a minimum haemoglobin content of 43 g.

The leukocyte content is less than 1.2×10^9 cells per unit and the average platelet content less than 20×10^9 cells per unit.

Methods of preparation

For the preparation of the component, the plasma and 20 to 60 ml of the buffy coat layer are separated from the red cells unit after centrifugation. Sufficient plasma is returned to the red cell unit to give Hct 0.65 to 0.75. Whole blood can be kept up to 24 hours in conditions validated to maintain a temperature between $+ 20°C$ to $+ 24°C$.

Labelling

The labelling should comply with the relevant national legislation and international agreements. The following information should be shown on the label or contained in the product information leaflet, as appropriate:

- the producer's identification;
- the unique identity number;
- the ABO and RhD group;
- the date of donation;
- the name of the anticoagulant solution;
- the name of the blood component;
- additional component information: leukocytes $<1.2 \times 10^9$; irradiated, etc. (if appropriate);
- the date of expiry;
- the volume or weight of the blood component;
- the temperature of storage;

- blood group phenotypes other than ABO and RhD (optional);
- that the component must not be used for transfusion if there is abnormal haemolysis or other deterioration;
- that the component must be administered through a 170-200 μm filter.

Storage and stability

As for whole blood.

Removal of buffy coat during component preparation reduces the formation of microaggregates.

Quality control

As for whole blood with the exceptions indicated in Table 6.

Table 6:

Parameter to be checked	Quality requirement (specification)	Frequency of control	Control executed by
Volume	250 ± 50 ml	1% of all units	Processing lab
Hct	0.65 to 0.75	4 units per month	QC lab
Haemoglobin	minimum 43 g unit	4 units per month	QC lab
Leukocyte Content/unit*	$<1.2 \times 10^9$	4 units per month	QC lab
Haemolysis at the end of storage	<0.8% of red cell mass	4 units per month	QC lab

*   These requirements shall be deemed to have been met if 90% of the units tested fall within the values indicated.

Transport

For red cells that have been stored in a refrigerator, validated transport systems should ensure that at the end of a maximum transit time of 24 hours the temperature should not have exceeded +10°C.

Transport by a non-refrigerated vehicle requires a cooled and insulated container.

Indications for use

Red cells, buffy coat removed (BCR) are used for replacement in blood loss and for the therapy of anaemia.

Precautions in use

Compatibility of red cells with the intended recipient must be verified by suitable pre-transfusion testing.

Red cells BCR are not recommended in:

- various types of plasma intolerance;

- exchange transfusions in newborns unless supplementary plasma is added;

- transfusion in premature infants and recipients with a risk of iron overload.

Side-effects

- circulatory overload;

- haemolytic transfusion reaction;

- non-haemolytic transfusion reaction (mainly chills, fever), but less common than after transfusion of red cells;

- alloimmunisation against HLA and red cell antigens;

- syphilis can be transmitted when red cells BCR has been stored for less than 96 hours at +4°C;

- viral transmission (hepatitis, HIV, etc.) is possible despite careful donor selection and screening procedures;

- protozoal transmission (e.g. malaria) may occur in rare instances;

- sepsis due to inadvertent bacterial contamination;

- biochemical imbalance in massive transfusion, e.g. hyperkalaemia;

- post-transfusion purpura;

- T.R.A.L.I. (Transfusion Related Acute Lung Injury);

- transmission of other pathogens that are not tested for or recognised.

Chapter 7: Red cells, in additive solution

Definition

A component derived from whole blood by centrifugation and removal of plasma with subsequent addition to the red cells of an appropriate nutrient solution.

Properties

The Hct of this component will depend on the nature of the additive solution, the method of centrifugation and the amount of remaining plasma. It should not exceed 0.70. Each unit should have a minimum haemoglobin content of 45 g.

The unit contains all of the original unit's red cells. The greater part of its leukocytes (about 2.5 to 3.0×10^9 cells) and a varying content of platelets depending on the method of centrifugation are retained, no effort having been made for removal.

Methods of preparation

The primary anticoagulant solution should be CPD. Most additive solutions contain sodium chloride, adenine, glucose and mannitol dissolved in water. Others contain citrate, mannitol, phosphate and guanosine. The volume may be 80 to 110 ml. Whole blood can be kept up to 24 hours in conditions validated to maintain a temperature between + 20°C to + 24°C.

After centrifugation of the whole blood unit the red cells and plasma are separated. After careful mixing with the additive solution the red cells are stored at +2°C to +6°C.

Labelling

The labelling should comply with the relevant national legislation and international agreements. The following information should be shown on the label or contained in the product information leaflet, as appropriate:

- the producer's identification;
- the unique identity number;
- the ABO and RhD group;
- the date of donation;
- the name and volume of the additive solution;
- the name of the blood component;

- additional component information: irradiated, etc. (if appropriate);
- the date of expiry;
- the volume or weight of the blood component;
- the temperature of storage;
- blood group phenotypes other than ABO and RhD (optional);
- that the component must not be used for transfusion if there is abnormal haemolysis or other deterioration;
- that the component must be administered through a 170-200 μm filter.

Storage and stability

The same storage conditions are applied as for whole blood and red cells.

Depending on the anticoagulant/additive system the storage may be extended up to the approved limit of the system.

Microaggregates are formed on storage.

Quality control

As for whole blood with the exceptions indicated in Table 7.

Table 7:

Parameter to be checked	Quality requirement (specification)	Frequency of control	Control executed by
Volume	to be defined for the system used	1% of all units	Processing lab
Hct	0.50 - 0.70	4 units per month	QC lab
Haemoglobin	minimum 45 g/unit	4 units per month	QC lab
Haemolysis at the end of storage	<0.8% of red cell mass	4 units per month	QC lab

Transport

For red cells that have been stored in a refrigerator, validated transport systems should ensure that at the end of a maximum transit time of 24 hours the temperature should not have exceeded +10°C.

Transport by a non-refrigerated vehicle requires a cooled and insulated container.

Indications for use

This component is used for replacement in blood loss and for the therapy of anaemia.

Precautions in use

Compatibility of this component with the intended recipient must be verified by suitable pre-transfusion testing.

Red cells in additive solutions are not recommended in:

- various types of plasma intolerance (may not concern units with a low plasma content unless IgA incompatibility is present);
- intolerance due to alloimmunisation against leukocyte antigens;

- exchange transfusion in newborns unless used within 5 days of donation, with the additive solution replaced by fresh frozen plasma on the day of use.

Side-effects

- Circulatory overload;

- haemolytic transfusion reaction;

- non-haemolytic transfusion reaction (mainly chills, fever);

- alloimmunisation against HLA and red cell antigens;

- syphilis can be transmitted when this component has been stored for less than 96 hours at +4°C;

- viral transmission (hepatitis, HIV, etc.) is possible despite careful donor selection and screening procedures;

- protozoal transmission (e.g. malaria) may occur in rare instances;

- sepsis due to inadvertent bacterial contamination;

- biochemical imbalance in massive transfusion, e.g. hyperkalaemia;

- post-transfusion purpura;

- T.R.A.L.I. (Transfusion Related Acute Lung Injury);

- transmission of other pathogens that are not tested for or recognised.

Chapter 8: Red cells, buffy coat removed, in additive solution

Definition

A component derived from whole blood by centrifugation and removal of plasma and buffy coat, and subsequent re-suspension of the red cells in an appropriate nutrient solution.

Properties

The Hct of the component will depend on the nature of the additive solution, the method of centrifugation and the amount of remaining plasma. It should not exceed 0.70. Each unit should have a minimum of 43 g of haemoglobin at the end of processing.

The unit contains all except 10 to 30 ml of the original units' red cells.

The leukocyte content is less than 1.2×10^9 cells per unit and the average platelet content less than 20×10^9 cells per unit.

Methods of preparation

The primary anticoagulant solution should be CPD. Most additive solutions contain sodium chloride, adenine, glucose and mannitol dissolved in water. Others contain citrate, mannitol, phosphate and guanosine. The volume may be 80 to 110 ml.

For the preparation of the component, the plasma and 20 ml to 60 ml of the buffy coat layer are separated from the red cells after centrifugation.

After careful mixing with the additive solution the red cells are stored at +2°C to +6°C.

Labelling

The labelling should comply with the relevant national legislation and international agreements. The following information should be shown on the label or contained in the product information leaflet, as appropriate:

- the producer's identification;
- the unique identity number;
- the ABO and RhD group;
- the date of donation;

- the name and volume of the additive solution;

- the name of the blood component;

- additional component information: leukocytes <1.2x109, irradiated, etc. (if appropriate);

- the date of expiry;

- the volume or weight of the blood component;

- the temperature of storage;

- blood group phenotypes other than ABO and RhD (optional);

- that the component must not be used for transfusion if there is abnormal haemolysis or other deterioration;

- that the component must be administered through a 170-200 μm filter.

Storage and stability

The same storage conditions are applied as for whole blood and red cells.

Depending on the anticoagulant/additive system the storage may be extended to the approved limit of the system.

Removal of buffy coat during component preparation reduces the formation of microaggregates.

Quality control

As for whole blood, with the exceptions indicated in Table 8.

Table 8:

Parameter to be checked	Quality requirement	Frequency of control	Control executed by
Volume	to be defined for the system used	1% of all units	Processing lab
Hct	0.50 - 0.70	4 units per month	QC lab
Haemoglobin	Minimum 43 g/unit	4 units per month	QC lab
Leukocyte Content/unit*	<1.2×10^9	4 units per month	QC lab
Haemolysis at the end of storage	<0.8% of red cell mass	4 units per month	QC lab

*   These requirements shall be deemed to have been met if 90% of the units tested fall within the values indicated.

Transport

For red cells that have been stored in a refrigerator, validated transport systems should ensure that at the end of a maximum transit time of 24 hours the temperature should not have exceeded +10°C.

Transport by a non-refrigerated vehicle requires a cooled and insulated container.

Indications for use

Red cells in additive solution, buffy coat removed are used for replacement in blood loss and for the therapy of anaemia.

Precautions in use

Compatibility of this component with the intended recipient must be verified by suitable pre-transfusion testing.

Red cells in additive solutions, buffy coat removed are not recommended in:

- various types of plasma intolerance (may not apply to units with a low plasma content);
- exchange transfusions in newborns unless used within 5 days of donation, with the additive solution replaced by fresh frozen plasma on the day of use.

Side-effects

- Circulatory overload;

- haemolytic transfusion reaction;

- non-haemolytic transfusion reaction (mainly chills, fever) but are less common than after transfusion of red cells in additive solution;

- alloimmunisation against HLA and red cell antigens;

- syphilis can be transmitted when this component has been stored for less than 96 hours at +4°C;

- viral transmission (hepatitis, HIV, etc.) is possible despite careful donor selection and screening procedures;

- protozoal transmission (e.g. malaria) may occur in rare instances;

- sepsis due to inadvertent bacterial contamination;

- biochemical imbalance in massive transfusion, e.g. hyperkalaemia;

- post-transfusion purpura;

- T.R.A.L.I. (Transfusion Related Acute Lung Injury);

- transmission of other pathogens that are not tested for or recognised.

Chapter 9: Red cells, washed

Definition

A component derived from whole blood by centrifugation and removal of plasma, with subsequent washing of the red cells in an isotonic solution.

Properties

This component is a red cell suspension from which most of the plasma, leukocytes and platelets have been removed. The amount of residual plasma will depend upon the washing protocol. The Hct can be varied according to clinical need. Each unit should have a minimum of 40 g of haemoglobin at the end of processing.

Methods of preparation

After centrifugation and maximal removal of plasma and buffy coat, the red cells are processed by sequential addition of cold (+4°C) isotonic saline and preferably refrigerated centrifugation.

Labelling

The labelling should comply with the relevant national legislation and international agreements. The following information should be shown on the label or contained in the product information leaflet, as appropriate:

- the producer's identification;
- the unique identity number;
- the ABO and RhD group;
- the date of preparation;
- the name and volume of the additive solution (if any);
- the name of the blood component;
- additional component information: leukocyte depleted, irradiated, haematocrit, etc. (if appropriate);
- the date and time of expiry;
- the volume or weight of the blood component;
- the temperature of storage;
- blood group phenotypes other than ABO and RhD (optional);
- that the component must not be used for transfusion if there is abnormal haemolysis or other deterioration;

- that the component must be administered through a 170-200 μm filter.

Storage and stability

During storage, the temperature of blood component should remain between +2°C and +6°C. The storage time should be as short as possible after washing and never exceed 24 hours when an open system has been used.

If a closed system and a suitable red cell solution are used, storage times may be prolonged subject to validation.

Quality control

As for whole blood, with the exceptions indicated in Table 9.

Table 9:

Parameter to be checked	Quality requirement	Frequency of control	Control executed by
Volume	to be defined for the system used	all units	Processing lab
Hct	0.65 to 0.75	all units	QC lab
Haemoglobin	minimum 40 g/unit	all units	QC lab
Haemolysis at end of the process	<0.8% of red cell mass	all units	QC lab
Protein content of final supernatant	< 0.5 g / unit	all units	QC lab

Transport

Transport is limited by the short storage time. Storage conditions should be maintained during transportation. Attention to strict control of temperature and time is required.

Indications for use

Washed red cells are only indicated for red cell substitution or replacement in patients with plasma protein antibodies, especially anti-IgA, and in patients who have shown severe allergic reactions in transfusion of blood products.

Precautions in use

Compatibility of the washed red cell suspension with the intended recipient must be verified by a suitable pre-transfusion testing.

As during the preparation the component may be transferred to another bag, measures should be taken to ensure the identification of relevant cross match samples and proper identification of each unit equivalent.

Side-effects

- circulatory overload;

- haemolytic transfusion reaction;

- alloimmunisation against HLA and red cell antigens;

- syphilis can be transmitted if the component is prepared from a blood unit which has been stored for less than 96 hours at +2°C to +6°C;

- viral transmission (hepatitis, HIV, etc.) is possible despite careful donor selection and screening procedures;

- protozoal transmission (e.g. malaria) may occur in rare instances;

- sepsis due to inadvertent bacterial contamination;

- transmission of other pathogens that are not tested for or recognised.

Chapter 10: Red cells, leukocyte-depleted

Definition

A component obtained by removing the majority of leukocytes from a red cell preparation.

Properties

The leukocyte count must be less than 1×10^6 per unit. Mean counts as low as 0.05×10^6 are achievable. Each unit should have a minimum haemoglobin content of 40 g.

Methods of preparation

Various techniques are used to produce this preparation including buffy coat depletion and filtration. The best results are currently achieved using a combination of both these methods. Whole blood can be kept up to 24 hours in conditions validated to maintain a temperature between $+ 20°C$ to $+ 24°C$.

A fully validated procedure must be established to determine optimum conditions for use of the leukocyte depletion method.

Pre-storage filtration is recommended, preferably within 48 hours after donation.

Labelling

The labelling should comply with the relevant national legislation and international agreements. The following information should be shown on the label or contained in the product information leaflet, as appropriate:

- the producer's identification;
- the unique identity number;
- the ABO and RhD group;
- the date of donation;
- the name of the anticoagulant solution or the name and volume of the additive solution (as appropriate);
- the name of the blood component;
- additional component information: leukocyte depleted, irradiated, etc. (if appropriate);
- the date of expiry and time of expiry, when required;
- the volume or weight of the blood component;

- the temperature of storage;

- blood group phenotypes other than ABO and RhD (optional);

- that the component must not be used for transfusion if there is abnormal haemolysis or other deterioration;

- that the component must be administered through a 170-200 μm filter.

Storage and stability

The same storage conditions are applied as for whole blood and red cells.

Removal of leukocytes before storage reduces the formation of microaggregates and the release of cytokines.

Red cells leukocyte-depleted, if filtered or prepared by other methods under which the system has been opened, have a storage life limited to 24 hours at +2°C to +6°C.

Quality control

As for whole blood, with the exceptions indicated in Table 10.

Table 10:

Parameter to be checked	Quality requirement	Frequency of control	Control executed by
Volume	To be defined for the system used	1% of all units	Processing lab
Hct	0.50 - 0.70	4 units per month	QC lab
Residual leukocytes*	$<1 \times 10^6$ per unit by count	1% of all units with a minimum of 10 units per month	QC lab
Haemoglobin	min 40 g/unit	1% of all units with a minimum of 4 units per month	QC lab
Haemolysis at the end of storage	<0.8% of red cell mass	4 units per month	QC lab

*   These requirements shall be deemed to have been met if 90% of the units tested fall within the values indicated.

Transport

Similar principles as for whole blood and other red cell components will apply. Attention to strict control of temperature and time is required where an open system of preparation has been used.

Indications for use

The same indications as for red cells apply. This component is indicated for patients with known or suspected leukocyte antibodies or whose transfusion requirement is likely to be ongoing to prevent alloimmunisation to leukocyte antigens.

This component is considered by some clinicians to be an acceptable alternative to CMV negative blood for prevention of CMV transmission.

As during the preparation the component may be transferred to another bag, measures should be taken to ensure the identification of relevant cross match samples and proper identification of each unit equivalent.

Precautions in use

Compatibility of this component with the intended recipient must be verified by suitable pre-transfusion testing.

Other components used in conjunction with red cells leukocyte depleted must also be leukocyte depleted.

Red cells leukocyte depleted are not recommended in:

- various types of plasma intolerance (may not apply to units with a low plasma content);
- exchange transfusion in newborns unless used within 7 days of donation.

Side-effects

- circulatory overload;
- haemolytic transfusion reaction;
- non-haemolytic transfusion reaction (mainly chills, fever), less common than after transfusion of whole blood or other red cell components;
- alloimmunisation against HLA (rarely) and red cell antigens;

- syphilis can be transmitted when this product has been stored for less than 96 hours at +4°C;

- viral transmission (hepatitis, HIV, etc.) is possible despite careful donor selection and screening procedures;

- protozoal transmission (e.g. malaria) may occur in rare instances;

- sepsis due to inadvertent bacterial contamination;

- biochemical imbalance in massive transfusion, e.g. hyperkalaemia;

- post-transfusion purpura;

- T.R.A.L.I. (Transfusion Related Acute Lung Injury);

- transmission of other pathogens that are not tested for or recognised.

Chapter 11: Red cells, cryopreserved

Definition

A component derived from whole blood, in which red cells are frozen, preferably within 7 days of collection, using a cryoprotectant, and stored at −60°C to −80°C or below based on the method used.

Before use the cells are thawed, washed and suspended in isotonic sodium chloride solution or additive solution for red cells.

Properties

A reconstituted unit of cryopreserved red cells is poor in protein, granulocytes and platelets. Each reconstituted unit should have a minimum haemoglobin content of 36 g.

Methods of preparation

Two principles are in general use for preparation of cryopreserved red cells. One is a high glycerol, the other a low glycerol technique. Both methods require a washing/deglycerolisation procedure.

Labelling

The labelling should comply with the relevant national legislation and international agreements. The label on the frozen units states:

- the producer's identification;
- the unique identity number;
- the ABO and RhD group;
- the date of preparation;
- the name and volume of the cryoprotective solution;
- the name of the blood component;
- additional component information: leukocyte depleted, irradiated, haematocrit, etc. (if appropriate);
- the date of expiry (and time of expiry when required);
- the volume or weight of the blood component;
- the temperature of storage;
- blood group phenotypes other than ABO and RhD (optional);
- that the component must not be used for transfusion if there is abnormal haemolysis or other deterioration;

- that the component must be administered through a 170-200 μm filter.

After thawing and reconstitution (washing), the year of expiry should be changed to the date (and time) of expiry, and the name and volume of the cryoprotective solution should be changed to the name and volume of the additive solution (if any). The temperature of storage should be changed accordingly.

Storage and stability

Red cells in frozen state
These should be constantly maintained at:

- −60°C to −80°C if stored in an electrical freezer when a high glycerol method is used;

- −140°C to −150°C if stored in vapour phase liquid nitrogen, when a low glycerol method is used.

The storage may be extended to at least ten years if the correct storage temperature can be guaranteed.

Thawed reconstituted red cells
The product should be stored at +2°C to +6°C. The storage time should be as short as possible after washing and never exceed 24 hours when an open system has been used.

Quality control

As for whole blood, with the exceptions indicated in Table 11.

Table 11:

Parameter to be checked	Quality requirement (specification)	Frequency of control	Control executed by
Volume	> 185 ml	all units	Processing lab
Hb (supernatant) *	< 0.2 g/unit	all units	QC lab
Hct	0.65 - 0.75	all units	QC lab
Haemoglobin	> 36 g/unit	all units	QC lab
Osmolarity*	< 340 mOsm/l	1% of all units with a minimum of 4 units per month. If less, each unit.	Processing lab
Leukocyte **	$< 0.1 \times 10^9$ cells/unit	1% of units with a minimum of 4 units per month. If less, each unit.	QC lab
Sterility	Sterile	1% of all units with a minimum of 4 units per month. If less, each unit.	QC lab

*   Final suspending solution

**   These requirements shall have been deemed to have been met if 90% of the units tested fall within the values indicated.

Since cryopreservation allows prolonged storage, serum and/or plasma samples obtained at collection should also be stored to enable future testing for newly discovered markers of transmissible diseases.

Transport

If transport in the frozen state is unavoidable, storage conditions should be maintained. Transport of thawed reconstituted red cells is limited by the short storage time. Storage conditions should be maintained during transport.

Indications for use

Cryopreserved red cells are indicated for red cell substitution or replacement. This component should only be used in special situations:

- transfusion of red cells to patients with rare blood types/multiple alloantibodies;
- red cells cryopreserved for at least six months are recommended for immunisation purposes, to allow retesting of donors;
- could be considered in some cases for autologous transfusion.

Precautions in use

Compatibility of the washed red cell suspension with the intended recipient must be verified by a suitable pretransfusion testing.

As during the preparation the component may be transferred to another bag, measures should be taken to ensure the identification of relevant cross-match samples and proper identification of each unit equivalent.

When processing in an open system, the risk of bacterial contamination is increased and therefore extra vigilance is required during transfusion.

Side-effects

- circulatory overload;
- protozoal transmission (e.g. malaria) may occur in rare instances;
- viral transmission (hepatitis, HIV, etc.), is possible despite careful donor selection and screening procedures;
- alloimmunisation against red cell antigens;
- sepsis due to inadvertent bacterial contamination;
- transmission of other pathogens that are not tested for or recognised.

Chapter 12: Red cells, apheresis

Definition

A component obtained by red cell apheresis of a single donor using automated cell separation equipment.

Properties

A typical red cell apheresis consists of one or two units of red cells collected from the same donor.

Depending on the method of preparation and the machine used, one of the possibilities with this technology is to prepare units of red cells with predictable, reproducible and standardised contents of red cells. Each unit should have a minimum haemoglobin content of 40 g. Depending on the method of preparation and the machine used, the platelet, leukocyte and plasma content may vary.

Donor selection

See Chapter 1: Selection of donors, B. Apheresis donors.

Method of preparation

Whole blood is removed from the donor, anticoagulated with a citrate-containing solution and red cells are harvested from it alone or simultaneously with other blood components (platelets, plasma) by the apheresis machine. The remaining blood components are returned to the donor. Either one or two units of red cells can be collected during a single procedure. During or after the procedure, a red cell storage solution is added. The volume of this storage solution may be between 80 and 120 ml, dependent on amount of red cells collected, collection haematocrit and storage haematocrit targeted. To reduce the number of contaminating leukocytes an additional filtration step may be included in the process.

Labelling

The labelling should comply with the relevant national legislation and international agreements. The following information should be shown on the label or contained in the product information leaflet, as appropriate:

- the producer's identification;
- the unique identity number. If two or more units are collected from the donor in one session, they should in addition be numbered Apheresis unit 1, Apheresis unit 2, etc.;

- the ABO and RhD group;

- the date of donation;

- the name of the anticoagulant solution or the name and volume of the additive solution (as appropriate);

- the name of the blood component;

- additional component information: leukocyte depleted, irradiated, etc. (if appropriate);

- the date of expiry (and time of expiry when required);

- the volume or weight of the blood component;

- the temperature of storage;

- blood group phenotypes other than ABO and RhD (optional);

- that the component must not be used for transfusion if there is abnormal haemolysis or other deterioration;

- that the component must be administered through a 170-200 μm filter.

Storage and stability

The same storage conditions are applied as for red cells. Removal of leukocytes before storage reduces the formation of microaggregates and release of cytokines.

If filtered or prepared by other methods under which the system has been opened, the storage time is limited to 24 hours at +2 °C to +6 °C.

Depending on the anticoagulant/additive system, the storage time may be extended to the approved limit of the system.

Quality control

As for whole blood with the additions shown in Table 12.

Table 12:

Parameter to be checked	Quality requirement (specification)	Frequency of control	Control executed by
Volume	to be defined by the system used	1% of all units	Processing lab
Hct	0.65 - 0.75	4 units per month	QC lab
Hct (if additive solution)	0.50 - 0.70	4 units per month	QC lab
Haemoglobin	minimum 40 g/unit	4 units per month	QC lab
Residual leukocytes* (if leukocyte depleted)	$< 1 \times 10^6$ per unit by count	1% of all units with a minimum of 10 units per month	QC lab
Haemolysis at the end of storage	< 0.8% of red cell mass	4 units per month	QC lab

*   These requirements shall be deemed to have been met if 90% of the units tested fall within the values indicated.

Transport

Similar principles as for whole blood and other red cell components will apply. Attention to strict control of temperature and time is required when an open system of preparation has been used.

Indication for use
Those listed for whole blood and other red cell components will apply.

When 2 units of red cells are collected in one procedure, the product is ideally suitable for one recipient.

If leukocyte depleted, this component is an acceptable alternative to CMV negative red cells for the prevention of CMV transmission.

Precautions in use

Compatibility of the red cells with the intended recipient must be verified by suitable pretransfusion testing.

Red cells: apheresis is not recommended in:

- various types of plasma intolerance;
- exchange transfusions in newborns unless supplementary plasma is added;

Furthermore the same precautions should be applied as with "Red cells" and if leukocyte depleted as with "Red cells, leukocyte-depleted".

Side-effects

- circulatory overload;

- haemolytic transfusion reaction;

- non-haemolytic transfusion reaction (mainly chills, fever), less common when leukocyte-depleted than after transfusion of whole blood or red cells;

- alloimmunisation against HLA (rarely after leukocyte depletion) and red cell antigens;

- syphilis can be transmitted when this product has been stored for less than 96 hours at +4°C;

- viral transmission (hepatitis, HIV, etc.) is possible despite careful donor selection and screening procedures;

- protozoal transmission (e.g. malaria) may occur in rare instances;

- sepsis due to inadvertent bacterial contamination;

- biochemical imbalance in massive transfusion; e.g. hyperkalaemia;

- post-transfusion purpura;

- T.R.A.L.I. (Transfusion Related Acute Lung Injury) unless red cells are washed;

- transmission of other pathogens that are not tested for or recognised.

Chapter 13: Platelets, recovered

Definition

A component derived from fresh whole blood which contains the majority of the original platelet content in a therapeutically effective form.

Properties

Depending on the method of preparation, the platelet content per single unit equivalent will vary from 45 to 85 $\times$ 10^9 (on average 70 $\times$ 10^9) in 50 to 60 ml suspension medium. Similarly, leukocyte content will vary from 0.05 to 1 $\times$ 10^9 and red cells from 0.2 to 1 $\times$ 10^9 per single unit equivalent, unless further measures are taken to reduce these numbers.

The amount of platelets in an adult "standard dose" of recovered platelets is equivalent to the amount obtained from 4 to 6 units of whole blood.

Methods of preparation

Preparation of platelet-rich plasma (PRP)

Principle: a unit of whole blood stored in conditions validated to maintain temperature between +20°C and + 24°C up to 24 hours, is centrifuged so that an optimal number of platelets remain in plasma and the number of leukocytes and red cells are reduced to a defined level. The key points of the method are:

- effectiveness of centrifugation defined as g $\times$ min;

- temperature of the blood during centrifugation must be standardised;

- disturbance of the component layers achieved by centrifugation must be avoided;

- in removing the supernatant plasma the flow should not be too rapid and the separation must be stopped at the level of 8 to 10 mm above the surface of the red cell layer.

Preparation of platelets from platelet-rich plasma

Principle: platelets in PRP are sedimented by hard spin centrifugation; the supernatant platelet-poor plasma is removed leaving 50-70 ml of it with the platelets; finally the platelets are allowed to disaggregate and are then resuspended.

Preparation of platelets from buffy coat

Principle: a whole blood unit stored between +20 °C to +24 °C for up to 24 hours is centrifuged so that blood platelets are primarily sedimented to the buffy coat layer together with leukocytes. The buffy coat is separated and further processed to obtain a platelet concentrate. Either single buffy coats or 4 to 6 pooled (blood group compatible) buffycoats are diluted with plasma or an appropriate nutrient solution. After careful mixing, the buffy coat or buffy coat pool is centrifuged so that platelets remain in the supernatant but red cells and leukocytes are effectively sedimented to the bottom of the bag. The key points of the method are similar to those mentioned for PRP.

Leukocyte-depleted platelets can be prepared by filtration, pre-storage leukocyte depletion is recommended (preferably within 6 hours after recovery). Careful optimisation of the centrifugation conditions allow leukocyte-depleted platelets to be produced by the buffy coat method.

A fully validated procedure must be established to determine optimum conditions for the leukocyte depletion method used.

In special circumstances, volume-reduced platelets can be prepared (see Chapter 21). Washed platelets can be prepared for patients who have had repeatedly adverse reactions after platelet transfusion. The same is true for patients with anti-IgA antibodies, where platelets from an IgA deficient donor are not available. Washing three times with saline or buffered saline will decrease concentration of proteins in the supernatant solution by more than 3 log. At the same time 10 - 20 % of platelets are lost. Platelets should be resuspended in additive solution. The washing technique should be validated.

Labelling

The labelling should comply with the relevant national legislation and international agreements. The following information should be shown on the label or contained in the product information leaflet, as appropriate:

- the producer's identification;

- the unique identity number. If platelets are pooled the original donations must -be traceable;

- the ABO and RhD group;

- the date of donation;

- the name of the anticoagulant solution or the name and volume of the additive solution (as appropriate);

- the name of the blood component;

- additional component information: leukocyte depleted, irradiated, virus inactivated, number of donations combined to make the pool, etc. (if appropriate);

- the date of expiry;

- the number of platelets (average or actual, as appropriate);

- the temperature of storage;

- that the component must be administered through a 170-200 μm filter.

Storage and stability

Platelets must be stored under conditions which guarantee that their viability and haemostatic activities are optimally preserved. Platelets can be stored in plasma or in a combination of plasma and an appropriate nutrient solution.

Plastic bags intended for platelet storage must be sufficiently permeable to gases to guarantee availability of oxygen to platelets. The amount of oxygen required is dependent on the number of platelets in the product. Generally, acceptable storage is obtained when the concentration of platelets is <1,5 × 10^9/ml and the pH of the platelet product stays continuously between 6.4 and 7.4 under the storage period used.

Agitation of platelets during storage must be efficient enough to guarantee availability of oxygen but be as gentle as possible. Storage temperature should be +20°C to +24°C.

Viability of platelets is preserved up to seven days under optimal conditions. However, more than five days' storage of platelets is not at present recommended unless a validated system has assured absence of bacterial contamination.

Quality control

Demonstration of the swirling phenomenon, based on light scattering by platelets of normal morphology in movement, may be carried out either as a separate quality control procedure or as a routine part of the issue and transfusion of this component.

Quality control requirements as for whole blood with the additions shown in Table 13.

Table 13:

Parameter to be checked	Quality requirement (specification)	Frequency of control	Control executed by
HLA or HPA (when required)	Typing	as required	HLA lab
Volume	> 40 ml per 60 × 10^9 of platelets	all units	Processing lab
Platelet Count*	> 60 × 10^9/single unit equivalent	1% of all units with a minimum of 10 units per month	QC lab
Residual leukocytes* *Before leukocyte depletion*			QC lab
a) prepared from PRP	< 0.2 × 10^9/single unit equivalent	1% of all units with a minimum of 10 units per month	
b) prepared from buffy-coat	< 0.05 × 10^9/single unit equivalent		
Residual leukocytes** *After leukocytes depletion*	< 0.2 × 10^6/single unit equivalent	1% of all units with a minimum of 10 units per month	QC lab
pH measured*** (+22°C) at the end of the recommended shelf life	6.4 to 7.4	1% of all units with a minimum of 4 units per month	QC lab

*	These requirements shall be deemed to have been met if 75% of the units tested fall within the values indicated.
**	These requirements shall be deemed to have been met if 90% of the units tested fall within the values indicated.
***	Measurement of the pH in a closed system is preferable to prevent CO_2 escape. Measurements may be made at another temperature and converted by calculation for reporting pH at +22 °C.

Transport

During transportation the temperature of platelet components must be kept as close as possible to recommended storage temperature and, on receipt, unless intended for immediate therapeutic use, they should be transferred to storage under recommended conditions. It is recommended that they be further agitated prior to use.

Indications for use

The decision to transfuse platelets should not be based on low platelet count alone. A mandatory indication may be considered to be the presence of severe thrombocytopenia, with clinically significant haemorrhage attributable to the platelet deficit. All other indications for platelet transfusion are more or less relative and dependent on the clinical condition of the patient.

After validated leukocyte depletion, this component is an acceptable alternative to CMV negative platelets for prevention of CMV transmission.

Precautions in use

Upon pre-storage pooling (either buffy coats or platelet suspensions) platelets may be stored for up to 5 days following donation unless a validated system has assured absence of bacterial contamination. If the pooling of platelets is performed after storage, platelets should be transfused as soon as possible but no later than 6 hours after pooling.

As during the preparation the component may be transferred to another bag, measures should be taken to ensure the identification of relevant platelet cross-match samples and proper identification of each unit equivalent.

RhD negative female recipients of child bearing age or younger should preferably not be transfused with platelets from RhD positive donors. If platelets from RhD positive donors must be used in these circumstances the prevention of RhD immunisation by the use of Rh-immune globulin should be considered.

Side-effects

- non-haemolytic transfusion reactions may occur (mainly chills, fever and urticaria). The incidence will be reduced by the use of pre-storage leukocyte depleted platelets;

- alloimmunisation, especially to the HLA and HPA antigens, may occur. When leukocyte-depleted platelets are used, the risk of HLA alloimmunisation is reduced, provided that other transfused components are also leukocyte depleted;

- syphilis can be transmitted;

- viral transmission (hepatitis, HIV, etc.) is possible despite careful donor selection and laboratory screening procedures. However, risks of CMV transmission can be reduced by leukocyte depletion;

- protozoal transmission (e.g. malaria) may occur in rare instances;

- sepsis due to inadvertent bacterial contamination;
- post-transfusion purpura may occur;
- T.R.A.L.I. (Transfusion Related Acute Lung Injury);
- transmission of other pathogens that are not tested for or recognised;
- Graft versus Host Disease in immune compromised patients.

Chapter 14: Platelets, apheresis

Definition

A component obtained by platelet apheresis of a single donor using automated cell separation equipment.

Properties

Depending on the method of preparation and the machine used, the platelet yield per procedure will vary from 200 to 800 $\times$ 10^9. Similarly, leukocyte and red cell contamination of the product may vary with the procedure and type of machine used. The method provides the ability to collect platelets from selected donors, to reduce risk of HLA alloimmunisation and for effective treatment of patients already alloimmunised. By reducing the number of donor exposures, the risk of viral transmission may also be reduced.

Methods of preparation

Whole blood is removed from the donor, anticoagulated with a citrate solution and platelets are harvested from it by the apheresis machine. The remaining blood components are returned to the donor. To reduce the number of contaminating leukocytes an additional centrifugation or filtration step may be included in the process.

With apheresis, the equivalent of platelets obtained from 3 to 13 whole blood units can be collected from a single procedure and can be divided into several standard units for transfusion.

Apheresis platelets can either be collected and stored in plasma, or in a combination of plasma and an appropriate nutrient solution.

Pre-treatment of donors with thrombopoietin is discouraged until the safety of such treatment has been further evaluated.

Washed platelets can be prepared for patients who have had repeatedly adverse reactions after platelet transfusion washed platelets may be indicated. The same is true for patients with anti-IgA antibodies, where platelets from an IgA deficient donor are not available. Washing three times with saline or buffered saline will decrease concentration of proteins in the supernatant solution by more than 3 log. At the same time 10 - 20 % of platelets are lost.

Labelling

The labelling should comply with the relevant national legislation and international agreements. The following information should be shown on the label or contained in the product information leaflet, as appropriate:

- the producer's identification;

- the unique identity number. When two or more units are collected from the donor in one session, they should in addition be numbered Apheresis unit 1, Apheresis unit 2, etc.;

- the ABO and RhD group;

- the date of donation;

- the name of the anticoagulant solution or the name and volume of the additive solution (as appropriate);

- the name of the blood component;

- additional component information: leukocyte depleted, irradiated, virus inactivated, etc. (if appropriate);

- the date of expiry;

- the number of platelets (average or actual, as appropriate);

- the temperature of storage;

- the relevant HLA and/or HPA type, if determined;

- that the component must be administered through a 170-200 μm filter.

Storage and stability

Platelets must be stored under conditions which guarantee that their viability and haemostatic activities are optimally preserved.

Platelet components to be stored more than 6 hours must be collected and prepared in a functionally closed system.

Plastic bags intended for platelet storage must be sufficiently permeable to gases to guarantee availability of oxygen to platelets. The amount of oxygen required is dependent on the number of platelets in the product. Generally, acceptable storage is obtained when the concentration of platelets is <1,5 × 10^9/ml and the pH of the platelet product stays continuously between 6.4 and 7.4 under the storage period used.
Improved platelet bags and optimised conditions for the preparation and storage of platelets may result in acceptable in vivo post transfusion recovery also at a higher platelet concentration and at pH values below 6.4 or above 7.4 as validated.

Agitation of platelets during storage must be efficient enough to guarantee availability of oxygen but be as gentle as possible. Temperature: +20°C to +24°C.

Viability of platelets is preserved up to seven days under optimal conditions. However, more than five days' storage of platelets is not at present recommended unless a validated system has been assured absence of bacterial contamination.

Quality control

Demonstration of the swirling phenomenon, based on light scattering by platelets of normal morphology in movement, may be carried out either as a separate quality control procedure or as a routine part of the issue and transfusion of these products.

Quality control requirements as for whole blood with the additions shown in Table 14.

Table 14:

Parameter to be checked	Quality requirement	Frequency of control	Control executed by
HLA or HPA (when required)	Typing	as required	HLA lab
Volume	> 40 ml per 60 $\times 10^9$ platelets	all units	processing lab
Platelet count*	> 200 $\times$ 10^9 /unit	1% of all units with a minimum of 10 units/month	QC lab
Residual leukocytes after leukocyte depletion*	<1.0 $\times$ 10^6 /unit	1% of all units with a minimum of 10 units/month	QC lab
pH** measured (+22°C) at the end of the recommended shelf life	6.4 to 7.4	1% of all units with a minimum of 4 units/month	QC lab

*   The requirements shall be deemed to have been met if 90% of the units tested fall within the values indicated. Residual leukocyte values much lower than these are obtainable with some apheresis machines.

**   Measurement of the pH in a closed system is preferable to prevent CO_2 escape. Measurements may be made at another temperature and converted by calculation for reporting pH at +22°C.

Transport

During transportation the temperature of platelet components must be kept as close as possible to recommended storage temperature and, on receipt, unless intended for immediate therapeutic use, they should be transferred to storage under recommended conditions. It is recommended that they be further agitated prior to use.

Indications for use

The decision to transfuse platelets should not be based on low platelet count alone. A mandatory indication may be considered to be the presence of severe thrombocytopenia, with clinically significant haemorrhage attributable to the platelet deficit. All other indications for platelet transfusion are more or less relative and dependent on the clinical condition of the patient. HLA and/or HPA compatible platelets may be useful in the treatment of immunised patients. It is recommended that these should not be obtained by apheresis of relatives of the patient or other HLA match individual who are potential haematopoietic progenitor stem cell donors.

After validated leukocyte depletion, this component is an acceptable alternative to CMV negative platelets for prevention of CMV transmission.

Precautions in use

RhD negative female recipients of child-bearing age or younger should not be transfused with platelets from Rh-positive donors. If platelets from RhD-positive donors must be used in these circumstances the prevention of RhD immunisation by the use of Rh-immune globulin should be considered.

The responsible physician should be informed if a unit of apheresis platelets which does not meet the recommended standards for platelets content must be issued for therapeutic use.

Platelets compatibility testing may be useful in the selection of platelets for transfusion to an immunised patient.

As during the preparation the component may be transferred to another bag, measures should be taken to ensure the identification of relevant cross-match samples and proper identification of each unit equivalent.

Side effects

- non-haemolytic transfusion reactions may occur (mainly chills, fever and urticaria). The incidence will be reduced by the use of leukocyte depleted platelets;

- alloimmunisation especially to the HLA and HPA series of antigens may occur. When leukocyte-depleted platelets are used, the risk of HLA alloimmunisation is reduced, provided other components used are also leukocyte depleted;

- syphilis can be transmitted;

- viral transmission (hepatitis, HIV, etc.) is possible despite careful donor selection and laboratory screening procedures;

- protozoal transmission (e.g. malaria) may occur in rare instances;

- sepsis due to inadvertent bacterial contamination;

- post-transfusion purpura may occur;

- T.R.A.L.I. (Transfusion Related Acute Lung Injury);

- transmission of other pathogens that are not tested for or recognised;

- Graft versus Host Disease in immune compromised patients.

Chapter 15: Plasma, fresh frozen

Definition

A component for transfusion prepared either from whole blood or from plasma collected by apheresis, frozen within a period of time and to a temperature that will adequately maintain the labile coagulation factors in a functional state.

Properties

This preparation contains normal plasma levels of stable coagulation factors, albumin and immunoglobulins. It should contain ≥ 70 IU Factor VIIIc per 100 ml and at least similar quantities of the other labile coagulation factors and naturally occurring inhibitors.

If fresh frozen plasma is to be used as source material for the preparation of fractionated products, reference should be made to the European Pharmacopoeia monograph on plasma for fractionation.

Fresh frozen plasma should not contain irregular antibodies of clinical significance.

Methods of preparation

a. **Whole blood**

Plasma is separated from whole blood collected using a blood bag with integral transfer packs, employing hard spin centrifugation, preferably within 6 hours and not more than 18 hours after collection if the unit is refrigerated. Plasma may also be separated from platelet rich plasma. Freezing should take place in a system that will allow complete freezing within one hour to a temperature below −30°C. If plasma is to be prepared from a single pack whole blood donation, adequate sterility precautions must be adopted.

Plasma may also be separated from whole blood, which immediately after donation has been rapidly cooled by special device validated to maintain the temperature between +20°C and +24°C and held at that temperature for up to 24 hours.

b. **By apheresis**

Plasma may be collected by manual or automated apheresis. The freezing process should commence within six hours of completion of the procedure in a system which allows complete freezing within one hour to a temperature below −30°C. Where use is made of a special device validated to rapidly cool the plasma to +20 °C and +24 °C and to maintain the temperature in that range, the plasma can be held at that temperature for up to 24 hours prior freezing.

c.   *Quarantine FFP*

This single donor FFP is released when the respective donor tests are negative for HBsAg, anti-HIV and anti-HCV in a blood sample collected after more than six months. After introduction of NAT-testing the reduction of the quarantine period could be considered.

Labelling

The labelling should comply with the relevant national legislation and international agreements. The following information should be shown on the label or contained in the product information leaflet, as appropriate:

- the producer's identification;
- the unique identity number. When two or more units are collected from the donor by apheresis in one session, they should in addition be numbered Apheresis unit 1, Apheresis unit 2, etc.;
- the ABO group;
- the date of donation;
- the name of the anticoagulant solution;
- the name of the blood component;
- additional component information: leukocyte depleted, irradiated, quarantined, virus inactivated, etc. (if appropriate);
- the date of expiry;
- the volume or weight of the blood component;
- the temperature of storage;
- that the component must be administered through a 170-200 μm filter.

After thawing, the date of expiry should be changed to the appropriate date (and time) of expiry. The temperature of storage should be changed accordingly.

Storage and stability

The stability on storage is dependent on the storage temperature available. Optimal storage temperature is at −25°C or lower. The following storage times and temperatures are permitted:

- 36 months at below −25 ° C;
- 3 months at −18°C to −25°C.

Quality control

<u>Table 15(a):</u>

Parameter to be checked	Quality requirement (specification)	Frequency of control	Control executed by
ABO, RhD∗	Grouping	all units	grouping lab
anti-HIV 1&2*	Negative by approved screening test	all units	screening lab
HbsAg*	Negative by approved screening test	all units	screening lab
anti-HCV*	Negative by approved screening test	all units	screening lab
anti-HBc* (when required)	Negative by approved screening test	all units	screening lab
Syphilis* (when required)	Negative by screening test	all units	screening lab
anti-HTLV I&II* (when required)	Negative by screening test	all units	screening lab

*   Unless performed on whole blood used as the source.

Table 15(b):

Parameter to be checked	Quality requirement (specification)	Frequency of control	Control executed by
Volume	stated volume ± 10%	all units	processing lab
Factor VIIIc	Average (after freezing and thawing): ≥ 70 % of the value of the freshly collected plasma unit	Every 3 months 10 units in the first month of storage*.	QC lab
Residual cells**	red cells: < 6.0 × 10^9/l leukocytes: < 0.1 × 10^9/l platelets: < 50 × 10^9/l	1% of all units with a minimum of 4 units/month	QC lab
Leakage	no leakage at any part of container e.g. visual inspection after pressure in a plasma extractor, before freezing and after thawing	all units	processing and receiving laboratory
Visual changes	no abnormal colour or visible clots	all units	"

* The exact number of units to be tested could be determined by statistical process control.
** Cell counting performed before freezing. Low levels can be achieved if specific cellular depletions are included in the protocol.

Transport

Storage temperature should be maintained during transport. Unless for immediate use, the packs should be transferred at once to storage at the recommended temperature.

Indications for use

Fresh frozen plasma may be used in coagulation disorders, particularly in those clinical situations in which a multiple coagulation deficit exists and only where no suitable virus inactivated stable product specific clotting factor concentrate is available.

Fresh frozen plasma may be used in the treatment of thrombotic thrombocytopenic purpura (TTP).

Its major use is as source material for plasma fractionation.

Precautions in use

Fresh frozen plasma should not be used simply to correct a volume deficit in the absence of a coagulation deficit nor as a source of immunoglobulins.

Fresh frozen plasma should not be used where a suitable virus inactivated specific clotting factor concentrate is available.

Fresh frozen plasma should not be used in a patient with intolerance to plasma proteins.

ABO blood group-compatible plasma should be used.

The product should be used immediately following thawing. It should not be refrozen.

Before use the product should be thawed in a properly controlled environment and the integrity of the pack should be verified to exclude any defects or leakages. No insoluble cryoprecipitate should be visible on completion of the thaw procedure.

Side-effects

- citrate toxicity can occur when large volumes are rapidly transfused;
- non-haemolytic transfusion reactions (mainly chills, fever and urticaria);
- viral transmission (hepatitis, HIV, etc.) is possible despite careful donor selection and screening procedures;
- sepsis due to inadvertent bacterial contamination;
- T.R.A.L.I. (Transfusion Related Acute Lung Injury);
- transmission of other pathogens that are not tested for or recognised.

Chapter 16: Cryoprecipitate

Definition

A component containing the cryoglobulin fraction of plasma obtained by further processing of fresh frozen plasma prepared from hard-spun cell free plasma and concentrated to a final volume of up to 40 ml.

Properties

Contains a major portion of the Factor VIII, von Willebrand factor, fibrinogen, Factor XIII and fibronectin present in freshly drawn and separated plasma.

Methods of preparation

The frozen plasma pack, still attached to other integral (or connected by a sterile docking device) satellite pack(s) and/or the primary blood pack, is allowed to thaw, either overnight at +2°C to +6°C or by the rapid-thaw siphon technique.

Following slow-thaw at +2°C to +6°C, the pack system is recentrifuged using hard spin at the same temperature, the supernatant cryo-poor plasma then being expressed on to the donor red cells or into a separate satellite pack. By either thawing or separation technique, some supernatant plasma is left with the cryoprecipitate to produce a final volume of up to 40 ml. The components prepared are then separated from each other using a secure, approved method for dividing the transfer tubing refrozen to the appropriate core temperature and held under appropriate storage conditions.

Alternatively, plasma obtained by apheresis may be used as the starting material, the final component being prepared by the same freezing/thawing/refreezing technique.

Virus inactivation and/or quarantine of this component is a requirement in some countries.

Labelling

The labelling should comply with the relevant national legislation and international agreements. The following information should be shown on the label or contained in the product information leaflet, as appropriate:

- the producer's identification;

- the unique identity number. When two or more units are prepared from plasma collected by apheresis in one session, they should in addition be numbered Apheresis unit 1, Apheresis unit 2, etc.;

- the ABO group;

- the date of preparation;

- the name of the blood component;

- additional component information: leukocyte depleted, irradiated, quarantined, virus inactivated, etc. (if appropriate);

- the date of expiry;

- the volume or weight of the blood component;

- the temperature of storage;

- that the component must be administered through a 170-200 μm filter.

After thawing, the date of expiry should be changed to the appropriate date (and time) of expiry. The temperature of storage should be changed accordingly.

Storage and stability

The stability on storage is dependent on the storage temperature available. Optimal storage temperature is −25°C and the following are permitted storage times and temperatures:

- 36 months at below −25°C;

- 3 months at −18°C to −25°C.

Quality control

As indicated in Table 15(a) with the following additions:

Table 16:

Parameter to be checked	Quality requirement	Frequency of control	Control executed by
Volume	30 to 40 ml	all units	Processing lab
Factor VIIIc	≥ 70 IU per unit	Every two months: a. pool of 6 units of mixed blood groups during first month of storage b. pool of 6 units of mixed blood groups during last month of storage	QC lab
Fibrinogen	≥ 140 mg per unit	1% of all units with a minimum of 4 units per month	QC lab
Von Willebrand Factor	> 100 IU per unit	Every two months: a. pool of 6 units of mixed blood groups during first month of storage b. pool of 6 units of mixed blood groups during last month of storage	QC lab

Transport

Storage temperature should be maintained during transport. The receiving hospital should ensure that packs have remained frozen during transit. Unless for immediate use, the packs should be transferred at once to storage at the recommended temperature.

Indications for use

Uses include:

a)   Factor VIII deficiency state (where a suitable specific clotting factor concentrate is not available);

b)   other complex deficiency states like disseminated intravascular coagulation;

c)   fibrinogen defects (quantitative and qualitative).

Precautions in use

The pack of cryoprecipitate should be thawed in a properly controlled environment at +37°C immediately after removal from storage and immediately before use. Dissolving of the precipitate should be encouraged by careful manipulation during the thawing procedure.

At low temperatures the plastic container may fracture and during thawing the pack should be carefully inspected for leaks, and discarded if any are found.

The pack should not be refrozen.

Side-effects

- non-haemolytic transfusion reactions (mainly chills, fever and urticaria);
- possibility of development of inhibitors to Factor VIII in the haemophiliac;
- viral transmission (hepatitis, HIV, etc.) is possible despite careful donor selection and screening procedures;
- sepsis due to inadvertent bacterial contamination;
- in rare instances, haemolysis of recipient red blood cells due to high titre alloagglutinins in the donor have been recorded;
- transmission of other pathogens that are not tested for or recognised.

Small pool preparations

In some situations, it may be desirable to pool up to 10 single-donor cryoprecipitate units. If this is carried out by an open technique, the pool should be used within 1 hour, and not refrozen for further storage. Appropriate labelling of the pool must ensure that its individual constituents can be traced without difficulty.

Chapter 17: Plasma, fresh frozen, cryoprecipitate-depleted

Definition

A component prepared from plasma by the removal of cryoprecipitate.

Properties

Its content of albumin, immunoglobulins and coagulation factors is the same as that of fresh frozen plasma, except that the levels of the labile Factors V and VIII are markedly reduced. The fibrinogen concentration is also reduced in comparison to fresh frozen plasma. Cryoprecipitate-depleted plasma should not contain irregular antibodies of clinical significance.

Method of preparation

Cryoprecipitate-depleted plasma is the by-product of the preparation of cryoprecipitate from fresh frozen plasma.

Viral inactivation and/or quarantine of this component is a requirement in some countries.

Labelling

The labelling should comply with the relevant national legislation and international agreements. The following information should be shown on the label or contained in the product information leaflet, as appropriate:

- the producer's identification;
- the unique identity number. When two or more units are prepared from plasma collected by apheresis in one session, they should in addition be numbered Apheresis unit 1, Apheresis unit 2, etc.;
- the ABO group;
- the date of preparation;
- the name of the anticoagulant solution;
- the name of the blood component;
- additional component information: leukocyte depleted, irradiated, quarantined, virus inactivated, etc. (if appropriate);
- the date of expiry;
- the volume or weight of the blood component;

- the temperature of storage;
- that the component must be administered through a 170-200 μm filter.

After thawing, the date of expiry should be changed to the appropriate date (and time) of expiry. The temperature of storage should be changed accordingly.

Storage and stability

The stability on storage is dependent on the storage temperature available. Optimal storage temperature is -25°C and the following are permitted storage times and temperatures:

- 36 months at below -25°C;
- 3 months at -18°C to -25°C.

Quality control

As indicated in Table 15(a) with the following additions:

Table 17:

Parameter to be checked	Quality requirement	Frequency of control	Control executed by
Volume	stated volume ± 10%	all units	processing lab

Transport

Storage temperature should be maintained during transport. The receiving hospital should ensure that frozen packs have remained frozen during transit. Unless for immediate use, the packs should be transferred at once to storage at the recommended temperature.

Indications for use

Cryoprecipitate-depleted plasma is indicated in TTP only.

Precautions in use

The routine use of this material is not encouraged because of the risk of viral transmission, and the general availability of safer alternatives.

This product should not be used in a patient with intolerance to plasma protein. Blood group compatible plasma should be used. The product should be used immediately following thawing: it should not be refrozen.

If cryoprecipitate-depleted plasma has been frozen after production, flocculation can occur upon re-thawing. Before freezing and after thawing, the pack should be carefully inspected for leaks.

Side-effects

- non-haemolytic transfusion reaction (mainly chills, fever and urticaria);
- citrate toxicity can occur when large volumes are rapidly transfused;
- viral transmission (hepatitis, HIV, etc.) is possible despite careful donor selection and screening procedures;
- sepsis due to inadvertent bacterial contamination;
- T.R.A.L.I. (Transfusion Related Acute Lung Injury);
- transmission of other pathogens that are not tested for or recognised.

Chapter 18: Platelets cryopreserved, apheresis

Definition

A component prepared by the freezing of platelets within 24 hours of collection, using a cryoprotectant, storing them at −80°C or below.

Properties

A reconstituted unit of cryopreserved platelets poor in red cells and leukocytes. The method provides the ability to store platelets from selected donors or for autologous use.

Method of preparation

Two methods are in general use for preparation of cryopreserved platelets. One is a DMSO (6% w/v), the other a very low glycerol (5% w/v), technique.

Before use the platelets are thawed and washed (or suspended) in autologous platelet poor plasma, in isotonic sodium chloride solution or suitable additive solution.

Labelling

The labelling should comply with the relevant national legislation and international agreements. The label on the frozen unit states:

- the producer's identification;

- the unique identity number; When two or more units are collected from the donor in one session, they should in addition be numbered Apheresis unit 1, Apheresis unit 2, etc.;

- the ABO and RhD group;

- the date of preparation;

- the name and volume of the cryoprotective solution;

- the name of the blood component;

- additional component information: leukocyte depleted, irradiated, virus inactivated, etc. (if appropriate);

- the date of expiry (and time of expiry when required);

- the volume or weight of the blood component;

- the temperature of storage;
- the HPA type (if determined);
- that the component must be administered through a 170-200 μm filter.

After thawing and reconstitution (washing), the year of expiry should be changed to the date (and time) of expiry, and the name and volume of the cryoprotective solution should be changed to the name and volume of the additive solution (if any). The temperature of storage should be changed accordingly.

Storage and stability

Platelets in the frozen state should be constantly maintained at:

- −80°C if stored in an electrical freezer;
- −150°C if stored in vapour phase liquid nitrogen.

If storage must be extended for more than one year, storage at −150°C is preferred.

Thawed platelets should be used immediately after thawing.

If short intermediate storage is required, the product should be stored at +20°C to +24°C with adequate agitation.

Quality control

As indicated in Table 14 with the following additions:

Table 18:

Parameter to be checked	Quality requirement	Frequency of control	Control executed by
Volume	50 to 200 ml	all units	Processing lab
Platelet count	> 40% of the pre-freeze platelet content	all units	Quality lab
Residual leukocytes (before freezing)	< 1.0 × 10^6 / dose	all units	Quality lab

Transport

If transport in the frozen state is unavoidable, storage conditions should be maintained during transportation.

Transport of thawed platelets is limited by the short storage time. Storage conditions should be maintained during transportation.

Indications for use

Cryopreserved platelets should be reserved for the provision of HLA and/or HPA compatible platelets where a compatible donor is not immediately available.

Precautions in use

- suitable HLA and HPA compatibility testing should be performed when required;

- toxicity of reagents used in its processing and cryopreservation e.g. DMSO.

Side-effects

- non-haemolytic transfusion reactions may occur (mainly chills, fever and urticaria);

- alloimmunisation, especially to the HLA and HPA series of antigens, may occur, but the risk is minimal;

- viral transmission is possible despite careful donor selection and laboratory screening procedures;

- protozoal transmission may occur in rare instances;

- sepsis due to inadvertent bacterial contamination;

- post-transfusion purpura;

- transmission of other pathogens that are not tested for or recognised;

- Graft versus Host Disease in immune compromised patients.

Chapter 19: Granulocytes, apheresis

Definition

A component consisting primarily of granulocytes suspended in plasma, obtained by single-donor apheresis.

Properties

The principal function of granulocytes is phagocytosis of bacteria.

Method of preparation

Leucapheresis by cell separator devices. Centrifugal flow methods, either intermittent or continuous, are used. Improved yields may be obtained by addition of a red cell sedimenting agent such as hydroxyethyl starch, low molecular weight dextran or modified fluid gelatine.

Pre-treatment of donors with corticosteroids and G-CSF is discouraged until the safety of such treatment has been further evaluated.

Labelling

The labelling should comply with the relevant national legislation and international agreements. The following information should be shown on the label or contained in the product information leaflet, as appropriate:

- the producer's identification;
- the unique identity number;
- the ABO and RhD group;
- the date of donation;
- the name of the anticoagulant solution and additive solutions and/or other agents;
- the name of the blood component;
- the date of expiry (and time of expiry, when required);
- the number of granulocytes;
- le temperature of storage;
- HLA type if determined;
- that the component must be administered through a 170-200 μm filter.

Storage and stability

This preparation is not suitable for storage and should be transfused as soon as possible after collection. If unavoidable, storage should be limited to 24 hours at +20°C to +24°C.

Quality control

Quality control requirements as for whole blood with the additions shown in Table 19.

Table 19:

Parameter to be checked	Quality requirement	Frequency of control	Control executed by
HLA (when required)	Typing	As required	HLA lab
Volume	< 500 ml	All units	Processing lab
Granulocytes	1×10^{10} per unit	All units	Processing lab

Transport

The unit should be transported to the user in a suitable container at +20°C to +24°C.

Indications for use

Can be used in severely neutropenic patients with proven sepsis while receiving adequate antibiotic therapy.

Precautions in use

As there is significant red cell contamination, compatibility testing is recommended.

Granulocytes should be exposed to an appropriate dose of ionising radiation before transfusion.

Side-effects

- non-haemolytic transfusion reactions may occur (namely fever, chills and urticaria);

- alloimmunisation to HLA and red cell antigens may occur;

- syphilis may be transmitted;

- there is a significant risk of transmission of latent viruses (CMV, EBV, etc.) to an immunosuppressed patient;

- viral transmission (hepatitis, HIV, etc.) is possible despite careful donor selection;

- protozoal transmission (e.g. malaria) may occur in rare instances;

- sepsis due to inadvertent bacterial contamination;

- post-transfusion purpura;

- accumulation of hydroxyethyl starch in multi-exposed patients;

- T.R.A.L.I. (Transfusion Related Acute Lung Injury);

- transmission of other pathogens that are not tested for or recognised;

- Graft versus Host Disease in immune compromised patients.

Chapter 20: Autologous predeposit transfusion

Several autologous transfusion techniques may be useful in surgery. They avoid the risks of alloimmune complications of blood transfusion, and reduce the risk of transfusion-associated infectious complications.

Autologous blood components can be obtained from pre-operative autologous whole blood donations in the weeks preceding surgery. In selected conditions, red cell or platelet concentrates can be collected using a cell separator: the equivalent of 2 to 3 red cell concentrates, or 4 to 10 standard platelet concentrate can be collected in a single procedure.

Autologous blood components obtained from pre-operative donations should be collected, prepared and stored in the same conditions as allogeneic donations. For these reasons, predeposit donations should be done in or under the control of blood establishments or in authorised clinical departments which are subject to the same rules and controls of this activity as blood establishments.

Acute normovolemic haemodilution is the collection of blood immediately before surgery, with blood volume compensation, leading to a haematocrit below 0.32, with reinfusion during or after surgery.

Red cell salvage during surgery is another means of autologous transfusion. Blood collected from operation site may be given back to the patient either after a simple filtration, or a washing procedure. These two techniques do not allow the storage of the collected blood. They are usually performed under the responsibility of anaesthesiologists and/or surgeons.

This chapter deals with autologous predeposit donations.

1. Selection of patients

1.1. Role of the physician in charge of the patient

In elective surgery situations where a blood transfusion is expected, the physician in charge of the patient, usually the anaesthesiologist or the surgeon, may prescribe pre-operative donations. The prescription should indicate:

- the diagnosis;
- the type and number of components required;
- the date and location of the scheduled surgery.

The patient is informed of the respective risks and constraints of autologous and allogeneic transfusion, and that allogeneic transfusion may also have to be used if necessary.

1.2. Role of the physician in charge

The physician in charge of blood collection takes the final responsibility for ensuring that the patient's clinical condition allows preoperative blood donation.

In case of contra-indication, the physician in charge of blood collection informs the patient and the physician in charge of the patient.

1.3. Informed consent

Patients should be informed:

- about the autologous transfusion procedure;
- about the biological tests, including virological markers, that will be performed;
- that allogeneic transfusion will be used in addition to autologous if needed;
- that unused units will be destroyed.

This information should lead to written informed consent being obtained.

In paediatrics, the information should be given to the child and the parents, and the parents should give a written informed consent.

1.4. Contra-indications of predeposit donations

Predeposit donation may be carried out safely in elderly patients. However, more careful consideration may need to be given in the case of a patient aged more than 70 years.

Children under 10 kg should not be included in a predeposit donation programme. For children between 10 and 20 kg, the use of volume compensation solutions is usually needed.

Any active bacterial infection is an absolute contra-indication.

In patients with haemoglobin concentration between 100 and 110 g/l, predeposit donation may be discussed according to the number of scheduled donations and the aetiology of the anaemia. No predeposit donation should be done in patients with haemoglobin concentration below 100 g/l.

It is recommended that patients positive for the following virological markers should not be included in a predeposit donation programme HBV, HCV, HIV and (when required) HTLV.

The presence of a cardiac disease is not an absolute contra-indication, and predeposit donation may be done, subject to the assessment of a cardiologist, if needed. However patients with certain unstable clinical conditions such as unstable angina, severe aortic stenosis, or uncontrolled hypertension should not normally be included in a predeposit donation programme.

1.5. Medications

Oral iron may be given to patients before the first donation and until surgery.

Any use of erythropoietin should comply with the product marketing authorisation.

2. Predeposit blood components preparation, storage and distribution

2.1. Blood typing and microbiological screening of autologous blood components

Blood typing and microbiological screening should be the same as the minimum required for allogeneic components.

2.2. Preparation of autologous blood components

The methods used for the preparation should be the same as for allogeneic components, but in a separate batch.

2.3. Labelling of autologous blood components

The labelling should comply with the relevant national legislation and international agreements. The label on the container states, in addition to the information valid for allogeneic blood components, the following:

- the statement: 'AUTOLOGOUS DONATION';

- the statement: 'STRICTLY RESERVED FOR';

- family name and first name, date of birth and identity number of the patient.

2.4. *Storage of autologous blood components*
Autologous blood components are stored under the same conditions as, but separate from, allogeneic components.

2.5. *Distribution and transfusion of autologous blood components*

Release procedures must include a confirmation of identity written on the components labels, on the prescription document and at the bedside.

Pretransfusion tests should be carried out as for allogeneic components.

Autologous plasma may be used as a volume expander until 72 hours after thawing, provided that it is stored in controlled conditions between +2°C and +6°C. Otherwise autologous components should be stored under the same conditions as their allogeneic counterparts but clearly separated from them.

Untransfused autologous blood components must not be used for allogeneic transfusion or plasma fractionation.

3. Records

Blood establishments and hospitals should both maintain the following records for every patient included in a predeposit autologous transfusion programme:

- the date and type of surgery;

- the name of the anaesthesiologist or the surgeon;

- the time of transfusion, specifying whether used during surgery or post-operative;

- the actual use of the prepared pre-operative autologous blood components;

- the concurrent use of peri-operative autologous transfusion techniques;

- the technique and the volume of autologous blood reinjected;

- the use of allogeneic blood components;

- the occurrence of any undesirable reaction related.

Chapter 21: Blood components for prenatal, neonatal and infant use

Specially designed blood components are required for prenatal transfusions or infant transfusions. The following aspects concerning neonates must be considered: (1) smaller blood volume, (2) reduced metabolic capacity, (3) higher haematocrit and (4) immature immunological system. All these aspects are particularly important in prenatal transfusions and for small prematures. There is significant risk of GvHD and CMV transmission in transfusion situations regarding small infants, a risk that is rapidly reduced with the increase in the infants' age.

There are specific national regulations for pretransfusion testing of blood groups and compatibility concerning neonates.

Methods of preparation, storage and administration of these components should be validated to ensure that the delivered potassium load is within acceptable limits.

1. Components for intrauterine transfusions

1.1. Red Cells for intrauterine transfusion

Definition

A component prepared from whole blood by removing leukocytes and part of the plasma as well as irradiating it.

Properties

The standard haematocrit (Hct) is 0.70 - 0.85. The leukocyte count must be less than 1×10^6 per unit. This level of leukocyte depletion prevents CMV transmission as effectively as the use of CMV negative blood. The product should be irradiated.

Red cells are prepared from O RhD-negative blood unless the mother has blood group antibodies which necessitate another blood group. The red cells should be antigen negative for any relevant maternal antibody.

To minimise the effects of potassium load the product should be used within five days from donation.

Methods of preparation

The standard way of preparing the product is to start from O RhD-negative blood and prepare leukocyte-depleted red cells and then irradiate the unit. Starting from filtered whole blood may offer another approach. The preferred method of preparation is prestorage leukocyte depletion.

Labelling

The labelling should comply with the relevant national legislation and international agreements. The following information should be shown on the label or contained in the product information leaflet, as appropriate:

- the producer's identification;
- the unique identity number;
- the ABO and RhD group;
- the date and time of preparation;
- the name of the anticoagulant or additive solution;
- the name of the blood component;
- additional component information: leukocyte depleted, irradiated;
- the date (of expiry and time of expiry when required);
- the volume or weight of the blood component;
- the haematocrit or the haemoglobin concentration;
- the temperature of storage;
- the relevant blood group phenotype, if the antibody is other than anti-D;
- that the component must be administered through a 170-200 μm filter.

Storage and stability

The component should be stored at +2°C to +6°C. The storage time should not be longer than 24 hours after concentration and irradiation.

Quality control

Quality control of the source material (red cells, leukocyte depleted) is stated in Chapter 10. Quality control of the final component is given in Table 21(a).

Table 21(a):

Parameter to be checked	Quality requirement (specification)	Frequency of control	Control executed by
Hct	0.70 - 0.85	4/month, if less each unit	processing laboratory

Transport

The storage conditions should be maintained during transportation.

Indication for use

Severe foetal anaemia.

Precautions in use

Monitor the speed of transfusion to avoid rapid intolerable changes in blood volume.

Side-effects

- circulatory overload;
- haemolytic transfusion reaction;
- syphilis can be transmitted;
- viral transmission (hepatitis, HIV, etc.) is possible despite careful donor selection and screening procedures;
- protozoal transmission (e.g. malaria) may occur in rare instances;
- sepsis due to inadvertent bacterial contamination.

1.2. Platelets for intrauterine transfusion

Definition

Platelets concentrate prepared from whole blood or apheresis technique is then processed further by removing leukocytes by filtration, irradiating it and concentrating platelets by removing part of the supernatant solution. A few apheresis systems may provide a leukocyte depleted component without a need for filtration or subsequent concentration.

In the case of transfusion of maternal platelets, these should be depleted of plasma and suspended in a suitable additive solution.

Properties

The component contains from 45 to 85×10^9 platelets (on average 70×10^9) in 50 to 60 ml of suspension medium. The component may be prepared from HPA compatible donor if necessary. The leukocyte content is less than 1×10^6 per unit. This level of leukocyte depletion prevents CMV transmission as effectively as use of CMV negative blood. The component is irradiated to minimise the risk of GvH disease.

Methods of preparation

The platelets should be leukocyte depleted, concentrated if necessary by removing part of the supernatant solution and irradiating the unit.

Labelling

The labelling should comply with the relevant national legislation and international agreements. The following information should be shown on the label or contained in the product information leaflet, as appropriate:

- the producer's identification;
- the unique identity number;
- the ABO and RhD group;
- the date and time of preparation;
- the name of the anticoagulant or additive solution;
- the name of the blood component;
- additional component information: leukocyte depleted, irradiated. Virus inactivated, plasma or supernatant reduced, etc. (if appropriate);
- the date of expiry (and time of expiry when required);
- the volume or weight of the blood component;
- the number of platelets;
- the temperature of storage;
- the relevant HPA type if necessary;
- that the component must be administered through a 170-200 µm filter.

Storage and stability

The component should be prepared as soon as possible after donation and used within 6 hours of any secondary concentration process. Secondary concentration by centrifugation should be followed by 1 hour resting period. Agitation of platelets during storage must be efficient enough to guarantee availability of oxygen but be as gentle as possible. Storage temperature should be +20°C to +24°C.

Quality control

Quality control of recovered platelets and apheresis platelets (the source material) is stated in Chapter 13 and 14 respectively.

Transport

Containers for transporting platelets should be kept open at room temperature for 30 minutes before use. During transportation the temperature of platelet component must be kept as close as possible to recommended storage temperature. On receipt it is recommended that the platelet be further agitated prior to use, unless required urgently. If stored, agitation is required at a controlled temperature of + 20°C to + 24°C.

Indications for use

Correction of severe thrombocytopenia which may be due to antenatal HPA alloimmunisation.

Precautions in use

- monitor the speed of transfusion to avoid rapid intolerable changes in blood volume;
- monitor the possible bleeding after puncture.

Side-effects

- viral transmission (hepatitis, HIV, etc.) is possible despite careful donor selection and laboratory screening procedures;
- syphilis can be transmitted;
- infection by inadvertent bacterial contamination of the component.

2. Components for neonatal exchange transfusion

Exchange transfusion is a special type of massive transfusion. Component(s) used must be fresh enough so that metabolic and haemostatic disturbances can be avoided.

In neonatal exchange transfusions one has to take into account ABO and Rh blood groups as well as other blood groups according to the maternal immunisation status.

Risk of CMV transmission and GvH disease must be prevented at least in the case of small weight premature infant and where the donor of the cells is an immediate relative.

2.1. Whole blood for exchange transfusions

CPD whole blood as defined in Chapter 4. Used within 5 days from donation. In case of anti-D immunisation O RhD-negative blood is used.

The product is leukocyte depleted and irradiated to prevent the risk of CMV-transfusion and GvH disease.

2.2. Reconstituted whole blood for exchange transfusion

Definition

To ascertain optimal safety and proper quality whole blood unit is reconstituted from fresh red cells and fresh frozen plasma. Blood group compatibility with any maternal antibodies is essential. The product is leukocyte depleted and irradiated to avoid the risk of CMV-transfusion and GvH disease.

Properties

The haematocrit (Hct) is 0.40 - 0.50.

The product is prepared usually from O RhD-negative red cells and AB RhD-negative fresh frozen plasma. If maternal antibody is other than anti-RhD red cells are selected so that it is compatible with the maternal antibody.

To minimise the effect of potassium load the product should be used within 5 days from red cell donation.

The product has the same metabolic and haemostatic features as fresh whole blood except very low platelet count. If the platelet count of the patient is very low, specific platelet transfusion should be given.

Methods and preparation

Leukocyte depleted red cells derived from blood group compatible donor are prepared as defined in Chapter 10. Supernatant containing additive solution and plasma are removed after centrifugation and AB RhD-negative fresh frozen plasma is added to reach haematocrit of 0.40 - 0.50. The product is irradiated and used within 24 hours since it is prepared in an open system.

Labelling

The labelling should comply with the relevant national legislation and international agreements. The following information should be shown on the label or contained in the product information leaflet, as appropriate:

- the producer's identification;
- the unique identity number (the original donations must be traceable);
- the ABO and RhD group of the red cells and the plasma;
- the date and time of preparation;
- the name of the anticoagulant solution;
- the name of the blood component;
- additional component information: leukocyte depleted, irradiated, haematocrit, etc. (if appropriate);
- the date of expiry (and time of expiry when required);
- the volume or weight of the blood component;
- the temperature of storage;
- the relevant blood group phenotype, if the antibody is other than anti-D;
- that the component must be administered through a 170-200 μm filter.

Storage and stability

The component should be stored at +2°C to +6°C. The storage time should not be longer than 24 hours after reconstitution and irradiation.

Quality control

Quality control of the source material (red cells, leukocyte depleted) is stated in Chapter 10. Quality control of the final component is given in Table 21(b).

Table 21(b)

Parameter to be checked	Quality requirement (specification)	Frequency of control	Control executed by
Hct	0.40 - 0.50	4/month, if less each unit	processing laboratory

Transport

The storage conditions should be maintained during transportation.

Indications for use

- Exchange transfusion of neonates.

- Massive transfusion in neonates and small infants.

Precautions in use

Monitor the speed of transfusion to avoid rapid intolerable changes in blood volume.

Side-effects

- circulatory overload;
- haemolytic transfusion reaction;
- alloimmunisation against HLA;
- syphilis can be transmitted;
- viral transmission (hepatitis, HIV, etc.) is possible despite careful donor selection and screening procedures;
- protozoal transmission (e.g. malaria) may occur in rare instances;
- sepsis due to inadvertent bacterial contamination.

3. Components for neonatal (small volume) transfusion

Besides the exchange and intrauterine transfusions small volume red cell, platelet and plasma substitution are also needed during the neonatal period. In fact babies in special care units are among the most intensively transfused of all hospital patients. Minimising the number of donor exposures is therefore a central aim in designing proper components and guiding the transfusion practice.

Therefore good practice is to divide a component unit into several sub batches and dedicate all the satellite units from a donation for a patient. Because fresh blood and red cells are used in intrauterine and exchange transfusions it is often thought that fresh blood is necessary for all neonatal transfusions. There is no scientific or clinical evidence to support this concept in case of small volume transfusions.

3.1. Red cells for paediatric use

Definition

A unit of buffy coat depleted red cells or leukocyte depleted red cells in additive solution are divided into approximately equal volumes of 25 - 100 ml.

Properties

Properties are the same as for red cells buffy coat removed or red cells in additive solution, buffy coat removed, or red cells leukocyte depleted.

Method of preparation

A unit of red cells, buffy coat removed (red cells: BCR) or red cells in additive solution, buffy coat removed (red cells: AS-BCR) or red cells, leukocyte-depleted is divided in equal volumes into 3 to 8 satellite bags by using closed or functionally closed system.

For small prematures and for some selected patients the red cell unit is to be leukocyte depleted and may be irradiated before or after dividing into satellite bags.

Labelling

The labelling should comply with the relevant national legislation and international agreements. The following information should be shown on the label or contained in the product information leaflet, as appropriate:

- the producer's identification;

- the unique identity number. When a blood component is split into two or more units, each sub-unit should be labelled with a unique sign in addition to the unique identity number;

- the ABO and RhD group;

- the date of donation;

- the name of the anticoagulant or additive solution;

- the name of the blood component;

- additional component information: leukocyte depleted, irradiated (if appropriate);

- the date of expiry;

- the volume or weight of the blood component;

- that the blood component must be administered through a 170-200 µm filter.

Storage and stability

The component should be stored at +2°C to +6°C. The storage time should not be longer than 35 days. If the component is irradiated, it should be used within 48 hours.

Quality control

As for the corresponding standard red cell product with the addition of the limits for the volume.

Transport

Storage conditions should be maintained during transportation.

Indications for use

- anaemia of prematurity;

- to replace the blood losses of investigative sampling;

- suitable for surgical replacement for infants and other children.

Precautions in use

Transfusion rates must be carefully controlled. The volumes of around 5ml/kg/h are regarded as safe.

Side-effects

- circulatory overload;
- haemolytic transfusion reaction;
- alloimmunisation against HLA and red cell antigens;
- syphilis can be transmitted;
- viral transmission (hepatitis, HIV, etc.) is possible despite careful donor selection and screening procedures;
- protozoal transmission (e.g. malaria) may occur in rare instances;
- sepsis due to inadvertent bacterial contamination.

3.2. Fresh frozen plasma for neonatal (paediatric) use

Definition

Fresh frozen plasma which is divided in equal volumes into satellite bags. Three to four of such bags are dedicated to one patient.

Properties

The same as for fresh frozen plasma (Chapter 15). National requirements may require use of plasma only from AB RhD-negative and positive donors.

Methods of preparation

Fresh frozen plasma is prepared otherwise by using the standard method (Chapter 15) but plasma is divided into small bags in equal volumes of 50 - 100 ml by using a closed system.

Labelling

The labelling should comply with the relevant national legislation and international agreements. The following information should be shown on the label or contained in the product information leaflet, as appropriate:

- the producer's identification;

- the unique identity number. When a blood component is split into two or more units, each sub-unit should be labelled with a unique sign in addition to the unique identity number;

- the ABO group;

- the date of donation;

- the name of the anticoagulant solution;

- the name of the blood component;

- additional component information: leukocyte depleted, irradiated, quarantined, virus inactivated, etc. (if appropriate);

- the date of expiry;

- the volume or weight of the blood component;

- the temperature of storage;

- that the component must be administered through a 170-200 μm filter.

Storage and stability

The stability on storage is dependent on the storage temperature available. Optimal storage temperature is at -25°C or lower and the following are the permitted storage times and temperatures:

- 36 months at below -25°C;

- 3 months at -18°C to -25°C.

Quality control

As for fresh frozen plasma (Chapter 15).

Transport

Storage temperature should be maintained during transport. The receiving hospital should ensure that packs have remained frozen during transit. Unless for immediate use, the packs should be transferred at once to storage at the recommended temperature.

Indications for use

Fresh frozen plasma may be used in coagulation defects, particularly in those clinical situations in which a multiple coagulation deficit exists and only where no suitable viral inactivated alternative is available.

Congenital deficiency of single clotting factors where no concentrate exists.

Precautions in use

Fresh frozen plasma should not be used simply to correct a volume deficit in the absence of a coagulation defect nor as a source of immunoglobulins.

Fresh frozen plasma should not be used where a suitable virally inactivated clotting factor concentrate is available.

Fresh frozen plasma should not be used in a patient with intolerance to plasma proteins.

Blood group-compatible plasma should be used.

Side-effects

- Citrate toxicity can occur when large volumes are rapidly transfused;
- Non-haemolytic transfusion reactions (mainly chills, fever and urticaria);
- Viral transmission (hepatitis, HIV, etc.) is possible despite careful donor selection and screening procedures;
- Sepsis due to inadvertent bacterial contamination;
- T.R.A.L.I. (Transfusion Related Acute Lung Injury).

3.3. Platelets for paediatric use

Recovered platelets or apheresis platelets as such or after leukocyte depletion can be used in the most paediatric patients. When preparing platelets for paediatric patients every effort should be made to minimise donor exposure.

Leukocyte depletion: To avoid excessive loss of recovered platelets filtration of a minimum of two such units is advisable. Some apheresis systems provide a leukocyte depleted component without a need for filtration or subsequent concentration.

Volume reduction: The clinical situation of a small child may necessitate the use of volume reduced platelets; Volume reduction to around 25 ml/unit causes in average 10% loss of platelets. The storage time is 6 hours after volume reduction.

Transport

The storage conditions should be maintained during transportation.

Indications for use

Severe thrombocytopenia of neonates of any cause.

Precautions in use

Monitor the speed of transfusion to avoid rapid intolerable changes in blood volume.

Side-effects

- circulatory overload;
- haemolytic transfusion reaction;
- alloimmunisation against HLA and red cell antigens;
- syphilis can be transmitted;
- viral transmission (hepatitis, HIV, etc.) is possible despite careful donor selection and screening procedures;
- protozoal transmission (e.g. malaria) may occur in rare instances;
- sepsis due to inadvertent bacterial contamination.

Labelling

The labelling should comply with the relevant national legislation and international agreements. The following information should be shown on the label or contained in the product information leaflet, as appropriate:

- the producer's identification;
- the unique identity number;
- the ABO and RhD group;
- the date of donation;
- the name of the anticoagulant or additive solution;
- the name of the blood component;
- additional component information: leukocyte depleted, irradiated, plasma or supernatant reduced, etc. (as appropriate);
- the date of expiry (and the time of expiry when required);

- the volume or weight of the blood component;

- the number of platelets;

- the temperature of storage;

- the relevant HPA type (if determined);

- that the component must be administered through a 170-200 µm filter.

Storage and stability

The component should be used within 5 days of collection, within 24 hours of any washing procedure and within 6 hours of any concentration process. Agitation of platelets during storage must be efficient enough to guarantee availability of oxygen but be as gentle as possible.

Storage temperature should be + 20°C to + 24°C.

Quality control

As for recovered platelets or apheresis platelets (Chapters 13 and 14), as appropriate.

PART D:
Technical procedures

Chapter 22: Blood group serology

General comments

The aim of any blood transfusion laboratory is to perform the right test, on the right sample and obtain the right results ensuring that the right blood component is issued to the right patient. It is essential to obtain accurate results for tests such as ABO/RhD grouping on the donor and patient, antibody screening and compatibility testing. In addition, there must be a reliable process in place for transcribing, collating and interpreting results to ensure that compatible and appropriate blood components are issued.

Errors at any stage of performing such tests can lead to incompatible or inappropriate blood being transfused with significant adverse health affects on patients. These errors can be due to either technical failure in serological testing or inadequate procedures leading to misidentification of patient or donor samples, transcription errors or misinterpretation of results. Haemovigilance data indicate that in some cases, a combination of factors contribute to error, with the original error being perpetuated or compounded by the lack of adequate checking procedures within the laboratory.

The implementation of a quality management system should help to reduce the number of technical and more often procedural errors made in the laboratory. These include quality assurance measures such as use of standard operating procedures, staff training, periodic assessment of the technical competence of staff, documentation and validation of techniques, reagents and equipment, procedures that monitor day-to-day reproducibility of test results and methods to detect errors in the analytical procedure.

The following pre-analytical, analytical and post-analytical procedures are required. For pre-analytical procedures, it is necessary to ensure and document that the reagents used are in-date and have been stored according to specifications. The donor samples used must be correctly labelled and suitable for the analysis to be performed. Appropriate performance checks should be carried out on equipment on a daily basis.

Analytical procedures must be performed according to the manufacturer's instructions.

1. Validation of reagents

The validation of reagents should detect deviation from the established minimal quality requirements (specifications). The Council of Europe has issued such requirements for blood grouping, and antiglobulin reagents. Summarised requirements are included in the tables of this chapter.

The blood groups reagents are considered as in vitro diagnostic devices and should be CE marked. An EU directive 98/79/EC classified the ABO RhD, Kell test serum, A B cells, HIV, HTLV, hepatitis B, C screening tests in list A. The manufacturer should have a full Quality System certified by an authorised body and submit an application containing all the control results for each reagent of these categories.

Moreover, it is assumed that an evaluation of quality is performed on samples before purchasing batches of commercial reagents. Prospective purchasers should expect potential suppliers to provide them with full validation data for all lot reagents. Each lot of reagent should be validated by the purchaser and the results should be as good as the specifications contained in the manufacturers monograph. Minimum potency standards for anti-A, anti-B and anti-D should be used in the assessment of blood grouping reagents.

Table 22(a): **Validation of reagents**

Parameter to be checked	Quality requirements	Frequency of control	Control executed by
Red cells reagents			
Appearance	No haemolysis or turbidity in the supernatant by visual inspection	each lot	Control Lab
Reactivity and specificity	Clear-cut reactions with selected reagents against declared RBC antigens	each lot	Control lab
ABO-typing reagents			
Appearance	No precipitate, particles or gel-formation by visual inspection	each new lot	Control lab

Parameter to be checked	Quality requirements	Frequency of control	Control executed by
Reactivity and specificity	No immune haemolysis, rouleaux formation or prozone phenomenon. Clear-cut reactions with RBC bearing the weakened expression of the corresponding antigen(s), no false reactions. (see also quality control of ABO- and Rh-typing)	each new lot	Control lab
Potency	Undiluted reagent should give a 3 to 4 plus reaction in saline tube test using a 3% RBC suspension at room temperature. For polyclonal reagents, titres should be of 128 for anti-A, anti-B and anti-AB with A_1 - and B cells; 64 with A_2 and A_2B cells	each new lot	Control lab
Rh-typing reagents			
Appearance	No precipitate, particles or gel-formation by visual inspection	each lot	Control Lab
Reactivity and specificity	As for ABO- typing reagents	each new lot	Control lab
Potency	Undiluted serum to give a 3 to 4 plus reaction in the designated test for each serum and a titre of 32 for anti-D and of 16 for anti-C, anti-E, anti-c, anti-e and anti-CDE using appropriate heterozygous red blood cells	each new lot	Control lab
Antiglobulin serum			
Appearance	No precipitate, particles or gel-formation by visual inspection	each lot	Control lab

Parameter to be checked	Quality requirements	Frequency of control	Control executed by
Reactivity and specificity	a. No haemolytic activity; no agglutination of RBC of any ABO group after incubation with compatible serum.	each lot	Control lab
	b. Agglutination of RBC sensitised with anti-D serum containing not more than 10-nanograms/ml antibody activity (0.05 IU/ml antibody activity).	each lot	Control lab
	c. Agglutination of RBC sensitised with a complement-binding alloantibody (e.g.anti-Jk^a) to a higher titre in the presence than in the absence of complement or agglutination of RBC coated with C3b and C3d.	each new lot	Control lab
Albumin			
Appearance	No precipitate, particles or gel-formation by visual inspection	each lot	Control Lab
Reactivity	No agglutination of unsensitised RBC; no haemolytic activity; no prozone or "tailing" phenomena.	each lot	Control lab
Protease			
Appearance	No precipitate, particles or gel-formation by visual inspection	each lot	Control lab

Parameter to be checked	Quality requirements	Frequency of control	Control executed by
Reactivity	No agglutination or haemolysis using compatible AB-serum. Agglutination of RBC sensitised with a weak IgG anti-D.	each lot	Control lab
	No agglutination of unsensitised RBC; no haemolytic activity	each new lot	Control lab
Saline			
Appearance	No precipitate, particles or gel-formation by visual inspection	each day	Control lab
NaCl content	0.154 mol/l (= 9 g/l).	each new lot	Control lab
pH	pH 6.6 - 7.6.	each new lot for buffered saline	Control lab
Low Ionic Strength Solution LISS			
Appearance	No turbidity or particles on visual inspection.	each lot	Control lab
pH	6.7 (range 6.5-7.0).	each new lot	Control lab

2. Quality control

The quality control procedures in blood group serology should be subdivided into controls for equipment, reagents and techniques. This classification is considered to provide clarity, in spite of partial overlapping, especially between controls for reagents and techniques.

Quality control of equipment

Equipment used in transfusion serology, in particular centrifuges, and automatic cell washers, water baths, incubators, refrigerators and freezers should undergo regular quality controls (Chapter 24). Equipment for automated blood grouping should also be controlled systematically, according to the manufacturer's instructions.

Quality control of reagents

Quality control procedures recommended in this section may basically be applied to reagents used for manual and for automated techniques. However, reagents for blood grouping machines may have special quality requirements and more detailed controls; the manufacturers of the equipment usually supply these.

Quality control of techniques

Provided that the quality of equipment and reagents fulfil the requirements, false results are due to the technique itself, either because of inadequacy of the method or - more often - because of "operational errors" as a consequence of inaccurate performance or incorrect interpretation.

Internal quality control

The quality control procedures recommended in this section are focused on the techniques but they will of course also disclose poor quality of equipment and/or reagents.

<u>Table 22(b):</u>   **Quality control for blood grouping**

Parameter to be checked	Minimal requirements for testing	Control samples	Frequency of control	Control executed by
1) ABO-grouping	Test twice in using two different reagents. Use of two different reagents*: monoclonal anti-A and anti-B from different clones; human antisera anti-A, anti-B and anti-A,B from different batches†.	One blood sample of each of the following types: O, A₁, B	Each test series or at least once a day provided the same reagents are used throughout	grouping lab

* When reverse grouping is undertaken, the two tests may be performed using the same reagents.

† If ABO and RhD blood group is already known, a single test is sufficient.

2) ABO reverse-grouping	Use of A and B cells.		Each test series or at least once a day provided the same reagents are used throughout	grouping lab
3) RhD – grouping	Testing twice in using two anti-D reagents from different clones or batches; use of the indirect anti-globulin test for weak D Confirmation in donors, where required. It must be ascertained that the system recognises the most important D variants (notably D variants category VI) as RhD positive†	One RhD- pos, one RhD-neg sample	Each test series or at least once a day provided the same reagents are used throughout	grouping lab
4) Rh and other blood group systems phenotyping	Use specific reagents	Positive control: RBC with tested antigen in single dose. Negative control: RBC without tested antigen.	Monoclonal antibodies and human antisera once a day	grouping lab
5) Antiglobulin testing tube technique	Washing the cells at least 3 times before antiglobulin is added	Addition of sensitised blood cells to negative test	Each negative test	grouping lab
6) Testing for high-titre anti-A and anti-B (in donors)	Use of A₁ - and B-RBC, Titration in saline or in antiglobulin test with plasma (serum) diluted 1:50.	Serum samples with an amount of immune anti-A and immune anti-B respectively above and below the accepted saline agglutination titre of anti-A and/or anti-B(16) Using antiglobulin test one control sample should give positive result and the other negative result	Each test series	grouping lab

7) Testing for irregular alloantibodies (in donors)	Use of antiglobulin test or other tests with the same sensitivity	Serum samples with known RBC-alloantibodies	Occasional input by the supervisor of the laboratory and participation in external proficiency testing exercises	grouping lab
8) Testing for irregular alloantibodies (in patients)	Use of at least the indirect antiglobulin test or manual or automated testing with equivalent sensitivity and homozygous RBC for the main clinically important antigens	as for 7	as for 7	grouping lab
9) Compatibility testing (including ABO and D-typing in donor and recipient RBC and test for irregular antibodies in patient serum)	Use of at least the indirect antiglobulin test manual or automated testing with equivalent sensitivity	as for 7	as for 7	grouping lab
10) Type and screen	Typing - as 1, 2, 3, and 4 with at least antiglobulin test, against a panel of cells chosen to provide homozygosity for important antigens	as for 7	each test series but at least daily	grouping lab

External quality assurance

The internal quality controls described above should be complemented by regular external quality assurance, i.e. participation in a proficiency-testing programme.

In external quality assurance, proficiency tests coded "normal" and "problem" blood samples are distributed from a national or regional reference laboratory to the participants, at least twice a year. The exercise can be limited to compatibility testing, since ABO-grouping, Rh-typing and -phenotyping as well as alloantibody detection will be automatically included. The proficiency test panel may consist of four to six blood samples, the participants being asked to test each RBC against each serum (or plasma) for compatibility. The panel should be composed in such a way that compatible as well as incompatible combinations occur. Asking for titration of one or two of the detected antibodies may complete the proficiency test.

In the reference centre the results are collated and accuracy scores determined. The results should be communicated to all participating laboratories (in coded or uncoded form, according to local agreement) in order to enable each laboratory to compare its own quality standard with that of a large number of other laboratories including the reference centre.

If no proficiency programme is available in a particular geographical area, the laboratory should arrange mutual proficiency testing with another laboratory. Although such an external quality control will not be as informative as participation in a comprehensive proficiency-testing programme, it will be a valuable addition to the internal quality control procedure.

Quality control of antibody quantitation

For practical purposes, RBC antibody quantitation is confined to the quantitation of anti-D. It is recommended that this be carried out by automated techniques rather than by manual titration, the test serum being assigned an anti-D value expressed in international units per millilitre after comparison with a curve derived from standard sera. All sera should be tested in duplicate as a minimum, and all national and in-house standards calibrated against the international standard for anti-D. Records should be kept of the data derived from processing the standard sera; these figures should show no more variance than two standard deviations. If automated technique is not available, manual titration by antiglobulin test is recommended.

Chapter 23: Screening for infectious markers

1.   General comments for all mandatory tests

The quality assurance of screening of donors for infectious markers is particularly important and implies both general and specific approaches. Only validated tests that have been licensed or evaluated and considered suitable by the responsible Health Authorities may be used. Screening test for infectious markers must be performed in accordance with the instructions recommended by the manufacturer of reagents and test kits.

An EU directive 98/79/EC classified the ABO RhD, Kell test serum, A B cells, HIV, HTLV, hepatitis B, C screening tests in list A. The manufacturer should have a full Quality System certified by an authorised body and submit an application containing all the control results for each reagent of these categories.

Blood establishments should validate all laboratory tests used for infectious disease marker screening to ensure compliance with intended use of the test. In addition proper validation demonstrates control, generates useful knowledge of the test and establishes future requirements for e.g. internal quality control, external quality assurance, calibration and maintenance of equipment and training of personnel.

There must be special emphasis on training of staff, assessment of staff competency, maintenance and calibration of equipment, monitoring of storage conditions of test materials and reagents, with documentation of all these actions.

Current tests for the screening of donations are based on the detection of relevant antigen and/or antibody and gene sequences. Tests are conventionally supplied in kits with the inclusion of negative and positive controls in each plate or run. The minimum performance requirement is the correct determination of these controls in accordance with manufacturer's instructions. It is further recommended that the tests include an external weak positive control in order to allow for statistical process control.

Initially reactive donations must be retested in duplicate by the same assay unless otherwise recommended by the manufacturer. If any of the repeat tests are reactive, then the donations are deemed repeatedly reactive and samples should be sent to the appropriate laboratory for confirmation and the donation may not be used for transfusion. In the event that the repeatedly reactive donation is confirmed positive, the donor should be counselled and a further sample obtained to confirm the results and identity of the donor. Ideally confirmatory tests should be as sensitive as and more specific than those used for screening. However, some screening tests are more sensitive than the available confirmatory tests. It is recommended that national algorithms be developed to enable consistent resolution of problems associated with discordant or unconfirmed results.

Algorithm infectious disease confirmatory testing

The following is an example of an algorithm:

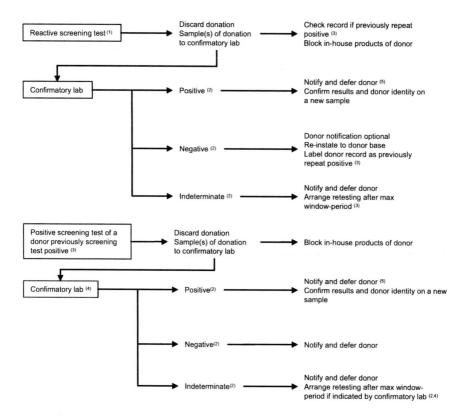

Conditions:

(1)
Eg. a repeat positive serological screening test or a positive NAT on a single donation.

(2)
Confirmatory lab is a certified / accredited medical microbiology reference lab, responsible for results, and may use tests at its discretion. Confirmatory lab is to be kept informed about the type of screening test used by the establishment, and is contracted to use tests at least as sensitive as screening test and if feasible based on other principles. Confirmatory lab is contracted to provide overall confirmatory test results or interpretation as follows: "positive", which means infected, "negative" which means not infected, or "indeterminate", which means a diagnosis cannot be established, the latter may include demand for follow-up testing. In case confirmatory testing is less sensitive than screening testing, the conclusion of confirmatory testing should read: "uncertain" (unless positive).

(3)   The establishment keeps a donor record allowing longitudinal recording of confirmatory lab test results as: screening test positive, confirmatory lab positive, negative or undeterminable.

(4)   Confirmatory lab is contracted to keep longitudinal records of unique donor ID linked to lab test results.

(5)   Refer donor to GP or specialist. Inform plasma fractionation centre(s) if plasma from earlier donation(s) has been issued. Inform hospital(s) to allow lookback if component(s) from earlier donation(s) have been issued.

The specific approach to quality of the screening must rely on the following categories of measures:

a.   Internal day-to-day quality control covering both reagents and techniques. Batch preacceptance testing (BPAT) of new batches of kits should be performed as an additional quality assurance measure;

b.   External quality checks, in particular confirmation of positive findings should be carried out by an appropriate laboratory;

c.   Occasional internal exercises, using a panel of sera which have been built up by comparison with standards available;

d.   External proficiency exercises, involving the testing of a panel of sera circulated to laboratories by an approved reference institution;

e.   All new techniques must be validated before implementation;

f.   Collection of representative data may be useful to monitor test performance.

It is recommended that repeatedly reactive rates and confirmed positive results of screening for infectious markers and epidemiological data be collected and monitored at least on a national level as part of a haemovigilance system. This will allow international comparisons to be made.

Some vaccinations may (temporarily) produce positive microbiology tests.

It should be noted that following hepatitis B immunisation, a transient positive HBsAg result may be obtained.

2.   Quality control of anti-HIV testing

All blood or blood components collected must be tested by an approved test which will reliably detect the antibody to HIV-1 (anti HIV-1) and HIV-2 (anti HIV-2) including outlying types (e.g. HIV-1 type O). The operating principles and requirements are as indicated in General Comments section.

The approaches currently used to confirm HIV infection consist of the use of a nationally established algorithm, which may include alternative ELISA's, Western blot or recombinant immunoblots. Tests for HIV antigen and the use of the NAT technology may be of value in the interpretation of uncertain anti-HIV test results. The positive confirmatory test should be repeated on a further sample taken between 2 and 4 weeks after the first.

Table 23(a):

Parameter to be checked	Quality requirement (specification)	Frequency of control	Control executed by
anti-HIV 1/2 screening sensitivity	detection of weak positive serum	each plate/run	screening lab

3.   Quality control of HBsAg testing

All blood or blood components collected must be tested by an approved test which will detect at least 0.5 IU/ml of hepatitis B surface antigen (HBsAg). The operating principles and requirements are as indicated in General Comments section. Confirmation of HBsAg reactivity must include specific neutralisation. The stage of infection of the donor may be determined by anti-HBc (total and IgM specific) and HBe antigen/antibody (HBeAg/anti-HBe).

Table 23(b):

Parameter to be checked	Quality requirement (specification)	Frequency of control	Control executed by
HBsAg screening test	detection of 0.5 IU/ml standard	each plate/run	screening lab

4. Quality control of anti-HCV testing

All blood or blood components collected must be tested by an approved test which will reliably detect antibody to hepatitis C virus (anti-HCV). The operating principles and requirements are as indicated in the General Comments section.

The approaches currently used to confirm HCV infection consist of the use of a national established algorithm, which may include alternative ELISA's and immunoblots. Sensitive tests for the detection of HCV antigen and genome may be of value in the confirmation of the infection status of the donor.

Table 23(c):

Parameter to be checked	Quality requirement (specification)	Frequency of control	Control executed by
anti-HCV screening sensitivity	detection of weak positive serum	each plate/run	screening lab

5. Quality control of syphilis testing

There is a continuing discussion over the need for a test for syphilis on blood donors, but the test may be used as an indicator of risk behaviours for sexually transmitted diseases and is still required by most countries. Most centres use either a cardiolipin test employing a lecithin-based antigen either manually or on blood grouping machines, or a test employing a variant of the *Treponema pallidum* haemagglutination assay (TPHA). An ELISA test is occasionally used. Positive syphilis screening results must ideally be confirmed by TPHA, fluorescent Treponema antibody test (FTA), or an immunoblot test.

Table 23(d):

Parameter to be checked	Quality requirement (specification)	Frequency of control	Control executed by
Lecithin-based reagent and TPHA reagents	detection of weak positive serum	minimum - start and end of run	grouping lab or screening lab

6. Quality control of malarial antibody testing

At present, only a few reliable and robust malaria antibody tests are commercially available. Any malarial antibody testing requirement requires integration within local approaches to donor history taking (see Chapter 1).

If malaria antibody testing is used to determine donor acceptance or rejection, the test employed should be shown to detect antibodies to the malaria types that are likely to pose a risk through transmission by transfusion.

Nucleic acid testing [PCR or other methods] cannot at present be recommended for use in blood donor selection. These methods may fail to detect a small number of parasites in a blood donation that is nevertheless sufficient to infect a transfusion recipient.

Confirmation of reactivity should be performed by a competent reference laboratory able to define the infectious state of the donor. Users need to be aware that assays may depend on the detection of heterotypic antibodies. Users must ensure that the assay detects antibody to the Plasmodium species prevalent in their donor panel.

The operating principles are as outlined in the General Comments section.

Table 23(e):

Parameter to be checked	Quality requirement (specification)	Frequency of control	Control executed by
Malaria antibody test	detection of weak positive serum	each run	screening lab

7.   Quality control of cytomegalovirus anti-(CMV) testing

Testing for CMV antibody is most commonly performed using ELISA and Latex particle agglutination test. The screening of donations for anti-CMV negativity will enable the formation of a panel of anti-CMV negative donations for use in highly susceptible patients.

Table 23(f):

Parameter to be checked	Quality requirement (specification)	Frequency of control	Control executed by
Anti-CMV screening test	detection of weak positive serum	each plate or run	screening lab

8.   Quality control of anti-HTLV testing

In any country where anti-HTLV testing has been implemented the operating principles and requirements are as outlined in the General Comments section. Selected donors may be tested by an approved test which will reliably detect antibody to human T-cell lymphotropic virus types I (anti-HTLV-I) and II (anti-HTLV-II).

The approach to confirmation is similar to HIV and includes nationally established algorithms as well as specific assays including immunoblotting and NAT. Sensitive tests for genome detection including typing may be helpful in defining the infection status of the donor.

Table 23(g):

Parameter to be checked	Quality requirement (specification)	Frequency of control	Control executed by
anti-HTLV I/II screening test	detection of weak positive serum	each plate/run,	screening lab

9.   Quality control of anti-HBc testing

In any country where anti-HBc testing has been implemented, the operating principles and requirements are similar to those indicated in General Comments.

Selected donors may be tested by an approved test that will detect antibody to hepatitis B core antigen (anti-HBc). The approach to confirmation should be dependent on a nationally established algorithm. Supplemental testing, such as anti-HBs, may influence local decisions about the acceptability of donors.

Table 23(h):

Parameter to be checked	Quality requirement (specification)	Frequency of control	Control executed by
anti-HBc screening test	detection of weak positive serum	each plate/run	screening lab

10. Quality control of HCV and HIV Nucleic Acid Testing (HCV- and HIV-NAT) in mini-pools

According to the requirements of the relevant European Pharmacopoeia monograph, all manufacturing pools for production of medicinal products derived from human plasma should be tested for HCV-RNA using a validated NAT assay which includes a suitable run control.

Table 23(i):

Parameter to be checked	Quality requirement (specification)	Frequency of control	Control executed by
HCV-NAT in mini-pools	detection of 5000 IU*/mL HCV-RNA per donation	internal control for each NAT reaction	NAT screening lab

* As defined by WHO standards

The Committee for Proprietary Medicinal Products (CPMP) recommends for HCV that a strategy of pretesting by manufacturers of mini-pools (of donations or of samples representative of donations) is encouraged in order to avoid the loss of a complete manufacturing pool and to facilitate tracing back to the donor in the event of a positive test result. Additionally some countries require screening of blood donations that are designed for the production of components for the use in transfusion by HCV- and / or HIV-NAT.

When such assays are used for release of blood components, the HCV- and HIV-NAT assay should be validated to detect 5000 IU / mL for HCV-NAT and 10 000 IU / mL for HIV-NAT (as defined for the single donation by WHO standards). For example, to achieve a sensitivity to detect 5000 IU / mL for HCV, if donations are tested in mini-pools of 100, 50 IU / mL should be detected with 95 % confidence by the assay. Each assay run should include an external run control (usually at 3 times the 95 % detection limit). This reagent must be reactive to every run. The external run control may be omitted if the test is licensed (CE marked) with other procedures to warrant robustness.

Chapter 24: Control of equipment

A. Environmental control

1. Routine laboratories

The same general principles apply as those suggested for permanent sessional venues. As set out in Chapter 2, section 1, the aim must be to provide a comfortable working environment for the laboratory staff and this must also comply with health and safety regulations. Bench design, as well as flooring, should be designed and constructed to be easy to clean. In addition to the control of temperature and humidity, excess noise must be avoided by the removal to a separate site of all excessively noisy pieces of equipment. Volatile and toxic materials must be handled in appropriate exhaust cabinets to avoid atmospheric pollution. A temperature monitoring device should be installed and regularly checked by the quality control.

2. Computers and electro-mechanical devices

These items of equipment may have special requirements such as a more precise atmospheric control or the provision of a non-standard or stabilised electrical supply. Such requirements should be checked with the manufacturer and secured before installation. Where special environmental control is necessary, temperature and humidity monitoring devices, including alarms, should be installed and validated. The readings should be taken by designated personnel at appropriate intervals and corrective actions taken when necessary.

These checks must be documented and traceable to an operator.

3. Blood processing laboratories

At transfusion centre level, blood component production may be either a closed process, as in the case of the separation of cells and plasma in a multiple bag system, or open, as in the case of washed red cells. A closed process may safely be carried out in the normal type of environment described for routine laboratories.

Open processes must be carried out under stricter environmental control either by the use of laminar flow cabinets or in the pressurised system of a suite of clean rooms provided with air passed into the inner cubicle through high efficiency particulate air filters.

B.   Validation of systems and equipment

Assessment of the performance of blood transfusion equipment must conform to Good Manufacturing Practice (GMP) and is mandatory on three specific occasions:

i.   on commissioning of new equipment, which must include full validation data by the manufacturer, design, installation, operational and process qualification;

ii. after any relocation, repairs or adjustments which may potentially alter the function of the equipment. Consideration should be given in the quality, safety and efficacy of any products processed before the repair or adjustment;

iii. if ever a doubt arises that the machine is not functioning properly.

Blood establishments should have a policy to assure proper maintenance of validated systems and equipment. It is necessary to establish a mechanism for assuring the adequacy of the calibration and monitoring programmes and ensuring that qualified personnel are available for its implementation. A calibration and monitoring plan should be used to define the requirements for establishing and implementing a calibration programme that includes the frequency of monitoring.

Trending and analysis of calibration and monitoring results should be a continuous process. Calibration and monitoring intervals should be determined for each item of equipment to achieve and maintain a desired level of accuracy and quality. The calibration and monitoring procedure should be traceable to a recognised international standard. The calibration status of all equipment that requires calibration should be readily available.

To ensure proper performance of a system or equipment a monitoring plan should be developed and implemented. The plan should take into account the criticality of the system or equipment, outline monitoring, user notification and problem resolution mechanisms. If an unusual event is observed, personnel should follow standard response described in the monitoring plan. The standard response should involve notifying affected personnel and initiating a resolution to the problem. Depending on the severity of the problem and the criticality of the system or equipment, a backup plan may need to be implemented to keep the process or system operating.

All critical equipment should have a regular, planned maintenance to detect or prevent avoidable errors and keep the equipment in its optimum functional state. The maintenance intervals and actions should be determined for each item of equipment. The maintenance status of each item of equipment should be available.

All modifications, enhancements or additions to validated systems and equipment should be managed through the blood establishment's change management procedure. It should be determined the affect each change has on the system or equipment and the degree of required validation. In addition to testing that evaluates the correctness of the implemented changes sufficient validation should be conducted on the entire system to demonstrate that portions of the system not involved in he change were not adversely impacted.

The competency of he blood establishment personnel to use and support systems and equipment correctly should be maintained. The training programme should be reassessed for any critical change in environment, equipment or process. Training records, including plans and protocols of the training status, ensure that training needs are properly identified, planned delivered and documented for maintenance of validated systems and equipment.

The availability of a supplier to maintain its activities related to a system or equipment has to be re-qualified on a regular basis to improve the partnership, to anticipate weaknesses in services or to manage changes in the system, equipment or supplier. The periodicity and the detail of the re-qualification process depend on the level of risk from using the system or equipment and should be planned for every supplier concerned.

A periodic review process should be established to assure that the system or equipment documentation is complete, current and accurate. A report of the review process should be produced. When deviations or problems are found actions should be identified, prioritised and planned.

C.   Reproducibility of results

A check of reproducibility is based on two principal concepts:

a.   the determination of accuracy of the equipment by the testing of a reference standard;

b.   the determination of the drift occurring during the routine day by testing of working standards at intervals.

Since examination of reproducibility usually implies that the test concerned is quantitative in nature, it follows that numerical values can be obtained for each type of control applied. Graphic plotting of the results of tests for accuracy and drift should be carried out so that a gradual deterioration in performance can be quickly identified and corrected.

Where a numerical value cannot be ascribed to the result of quality control tests, reproducibility can best be assessed by the inclusion in the schedule of testing of appropriate strong and weak positive controls at regular intervals.

Proper education of the personnel using blood transfusion laboratory equipment is essential. The staff must know not only how the control tests are to be done, but why they must be done, and they should be fully instructed not only in the performance of quality control tests but in the rapid detection of departures from the norm. In almost every case, normal functioning of the machine is defined by the manufacturer and confirmed at assessment on installation. Meticulous charting of quality control results preferably combined with statistical process controls will be the best methods of quick recognition of deterioration in function.

Table 24 lists some of the equipment used routinely in blood transfusion practice and the minimum requirements for their control. Other items of equipment, for example automated blood grouping machines, automated blood processing systems, etc. require the design of specific quality control procedures.

Table 24:

Equipment	Method of control	Frequency of control	Control executed by
Blood bag refrigerator, cold room, Freezer containing transfusates	Graphic recorder plus independent audible and visual alarm for appropriate high and low temperature parameters	daily	technician
Laboratory refrigerator, Laboratory freezer, incubators, water baths	(a) Thermometer	daily	technician
	(b) Precision thermometer	every 6 months	technician
Blood bag centrifuge	Precision RPM meter plus stopwatch to control speed, acceleration and retardation	at least once a year	engineering
	Temperature	daily	technician
Table centrifuge	RPM meter plus stopwatch to control speed, acceleration and retardation	occasionally	technician
Antiglobulin test automatic washer	Anti-D sensitised cells	every run	technician
Haemoglobin photometer	Calibration standard Hb quality control Sample	Daily monthly	technician

Equipment	Method of control	Frequency of control	Control executed by
Cell counters	Calibration: reference sample.	Daily	technician
	Drift: working standard		technician
Automatic pipettes	Dye- or isotope-labelled protein	at least once a year	technician
Balance	Analytical-control Weights 5 mg - 100 g	every 6 months or after each location change	technician
	Preparative control weights 100 mg - 100 g		
pH meter	Control solutions pH 4-7, 7-10	each time of use	technician
Platelet agitator	Thermometer	daily	technician
	Frequency of agitation	monthly	technician
Laminar flow hood and sterile area filters	Air pressure meter	daily	user
	Particle counter	tri-monthly	micro-biologist
	Bacteriological plates	monthly	micro-biologist
Blood mixer (swing)	Control weighing and mixing	bi-monthly	engineering
Spring balance for bags	Control weighing	monthly	engineering
Sterile connecting device	a) Tensile control by hand and visual control*	every 6 months	Engineering
	b) Standardised tensile strength or pressure test		
Blood transport container	In the absence of a validated transport system, minimum/maximum thermometer or a temperature recording device	every time of use (on receipt)	Technician

---

* Check for leaks [escaping fluid or air bubbles (under water)] by applying pressure to the tubing on both sides of the weld.

Chapter 25: Data processing systems

A.   Introduction

Electronic data processing systems are being used increasingly in blood centres for information management and storage and as tools for operational decision-making and control. Because these uses are critical to product and quality, these systems must be fully validated to ensure that they meet predetermined specifications for their functions, that they correctly preserve data integrity, and that their use is properly integrated into the centre's operating procedures. The developers of computer systems used in blood centres should follow established principles of software engineering design to develop, document and validate all source codes. Additional validation in the blood centre, at a minimum, should include provision of a written description of the system elements and their functions, and on-line performance testing of the system under at least limiting and boundary conditions. A record should be kept of the validation testing.

B.   Defining the system

A system includes people, machines and methods organised to accomplish a set of specific functions. A blood establishment's computerised system includes: hardware, software, peripheral devices, personnel, and documentation (e.g. manuals and Standard Operating Procedures, SOPs). To define the system, the user, in co-operation with the vendor or developer, should generate a written description of the system, the functions that it is designed to perform and all human interactions. The documentation should be current, accurate and as detailed as necessary to ensure proper operation of the system. The documentation should include:

1. a detailed specification of the hardware, software and peripheral devices, including their environmental requirements and limitations;

2. diagrams or flow charts of the system's operation describing all component interfaces, and all database structures, e.g. file sizes, input and output formats, etc.;

3. standard operating procedures (SOPs) defining when and how the system is used. In particular, SOPs should address all manual and automated interactions with the system including:

    a. routine, maintenance and diagnostic procedures;

    b. "work arounds" for system limitations;

    c. procedures for handling errors and disasters;

4. training manuals, materials and procedures.

C.   Testing of the system by the user

The purpose of user testing is to demonstrate that the system is correctly performing all its specified functions in its real world environment. Testing should be part of system installation. Testing also should be performed after any system modifications to ensure that the changes did not cause any unintended results. Testing should follow a written plan based on an expert assessment of the risks inherent in the system and their potential impact on the quality of blood products. The types of risk to consider include inadequate system design, errors that may occur in use, and loss or compromise of data. Testing may involve the whole system or only components. The following types of basic testing should be conducted:

1. Functional testing of components

The system components are presented with all types of expected interaction including normal value, boundary, invalid and special case inputs. The system should produce the correct outputs, including error messages by control programs. It is useful to perform this testing in parallel with a reference or standard system.

2. Environmental testing

In the actual operating environment, functional tests are performed to demonstrate that:

a. the systems work properly with its hardware;

b. applications software performs properly with the operating system software;

c. proper information passes correctly through system interfaces.

D.   Maintenance of the system

Maintenance activities apply to all elements of the system including hardware, software, peripheral devices, standard operating procedures and training. Maintenance activities include prevention, emergency management and quality assurance audits. At a minimum:

1. Vendor's recommendations should be followed for periodic use of utility and diagnostic software programs to test system integrity;

2. The database should be checked periodically to identify and remove unwanted data such as duplicate records, and to ensure that data entries

are accurate and properly stored. Manual entry of critical data requires independent verification by a second authorised person.

3. Security of the database should be maintained by:

    a. periodically rearranging electronic passwords (without re-use) and by removing unnecessary or outdated access;

    b. creating records of all data changes including a retained record of the previous data;

    c. the appropriate use of programs to detect computer viruses.

4. Data should be archived periodically using a long-term stable medium, and placed "off-site". Such archives should be challenged at least annually to verify data retrieval;

5. Procedures should be defined for:

    a. investigation and correction of discrepancies in the database; and

    b. corrective actions to be taken when validation testing yields unexpected results.

E.   Quality assurance

The quality assurance programme should exercise oversight of the electronic data processing systems that affect product quality. At a minimum, such oversight should include:

1. assuring the ongoing accuracy and completeness of all documentation on equipment, software maintenance, and operator training;

2. performing audits periodically to verify proper accomplishment of all performance tests, routine maintenance, change procedures, data integrity checks, error investigations, and operator competency evaluations.

Chapter 26: Record keeping

With records of results of quality control procedures a distinction should be made between records of results which may require prompt or almost immediate correction, and records of results which can only be evaluated statistically or by summing up over a certain period.

International rules and national laws on data protection have to be taken into consideration.

Examples of the former are given throughout the preceding chapters. Most typical examples are those where a quality control procedure is prescribed for each unit of a blood product or for each laboratory procedure.

Examples of the latter records (summary records) are given below. The director of the transfusion service or a specially designated person should evaluate statistical variations from the usual pattern or from given normal values. Evaluation may take place monthly or quarterly, and annually.

- Rejection or deferral of blood donors (numbers, reasons).
- Donor reactions (numbers, sex, age, reaction category).
- Unsatisfactory donations (numbers, category).
- Positive tests for infectious markers (numbers, specific, false).
- Discarded units of blood and blood components (numbers, categories, reasons).
- Outdating of units of blood and blood components (for each category, the outdating as a percentage of the number of usable units).
- Transfusion complications (numbers, category) including transfusion transmitted infection.
- External complaints (number, origin, category).
- Clerical errors (numbers, category).

There are a number of other records which are important in transfusion centres but which do not deal directly with quality control. Examples are: routine working documents, blood group documents for patients and donors, the proportion of cross-matched units to used (transfused) units of blood products, statistics of issue and return of blood units, etc. Many of these records are mainly used for administrative or organisational purposes.

It is essential that the recording system ensures a continuity of documentation of all procedures performed, from the blood donor to the recipient, i.e. each significant step should be recorded in a manner that permits tracing in either direction of a product or procedure from the first step to final disposition.

Specific consideration must be given to the ability to determine rapidly:

- each patient's history of transfusion including the reason for transfusion and the record of all components;

- the identity of the donors;

- each donor's history of donation;

- the final disposition (including the identity of the recipient) of all components from every donation.

Records of quality control procedures must include identification of the person(s) performing the tests or procedures. Any corrective action taken must also be recorded. If corrections in records are necessary, the original recording must not be obliterated, but must remain legible.

The manual entry of critical data such as laboratory tests results should require independent verification by a second authorised person.

Records of quality control procedures should be signed by the supervisor.

Records should be kept for a period according to local or national requirements. It is considered that the retention period should be at least fifteen years.

Retention of samples

Retention of donor samples for a period of time may provide useful information. The provision of such systems is contingent on the availability of adequate human and financial resources.

Chapter 27: Statistical process control

Introduction

Statistical Process Control (SPC) is a tool which enables an organisation to detect change in the process and procedures which it carries out, monitoring collected data over a period of time in a standardised fashion. SPC became mandatory in 2005 for blood establishments in the EU (Directive 2004/33/EC), and has been implemented in other industries. Consequently, methods and standards for application of SPC to Quality Assurance of blood components should be further developed. The technique can be applied to all activities in a blood centre, administrative and clerical as well as scientific and technical. It is important to prioritise the processes to which it will be applied due to the amount of work involved. The most valuable uses currently would be in monitoring the performance of testing of infectious markers and leukocyte depletion. SPC is one of the few methods by which it can be shown that an improvement to a process has achieved the desired result, and enables decision-making to be placed on a much more rational and scientific basis.

Feedback to the staff on their performance is essential for continuing quality.

Implementation of SPC

Alongside all other aspects of Quality, implementation of SPC demands understanding and commitment on the part of the management of the centre. It must be included in the Quality Policy of the centre, and a training programme introduced for senior management as well as operational staff. Plans must be made for data collection, including of charts, and all matters dealing with changes detected in the process, especially sudden "out-of-control" situations. Regular review of processes against charted data should take place, with the specific objective of improvement on a continuous basis.

Strategy for statistical sampling

As far as possible, the number and frequency of products sampled for quality control and the number of test failures per sample that will trigger an appropriate response (e.g. investigation, or revalidation of materials and procedures) should be based on the following considerations:

a)   Tolerance of failure

A "target failure rate" should be established as the failure rate that should not be exceeded. This will assure that monitoring of aspects of quality is continuous and that a failure rate exceeding target values will trigger appropriate corrective action.

b)   Confidence level

A confidence level should be set for detection of an actual failure rate which lies above the "target failure rate".

Determining that the actual failure lies above the "target failure rate" should be estimated using a valid method of statistical analysis.

Frequency of Control Sampling

A number of challenges arise in framing statistically based quality control testing programs for labile blood components. Due to the complexity of the issues, blood establishments should consult statistical experts when designing process control systems. The issues include the very large variation in volume of production at different blood establishments, the need to minimise product losses through testing at small centres, the very low expected rate of non-conformance for some processes, and the number of discrete conditions that arise in manufacture of otherwise similar products (e.g. number of sites, operators and work shifts; different collection and processing systems and equipment; use of multiple reagent lots; alternative preparation times and temperatures; etc.) Additionally, in many cases, the medical basis for currently accepted quality standards has not been established rigorously, making it difficult to determine the level of deviation from the expected rate of conformance that can be tolerated. Nevertheless, to implement statistical process control, the blood establishment needs to establish the "target rate" of failure that should not be exceeded for each control test. Additionally, it is desirable that the criterion for determining non-conformance should have at least a power of 80% to detect the "target rate" of failure, while giving a false positive result in fewer than 5% of determinations.

Consideration also must be given to the strategy for representative sampling of units for control testing. Because similar products are prepared under a variety of conditions, it is important that the sample set should include representative units prepared in all possible ways. Sampling may need to be stratified accordingly (i.e. to include a minimum number of samples from each condition). Additionally, there may be merit either in a strategy of random sampling over time, or in a strategy to sample sequential units (e.g. first set of some number of units prepared in each month.) Random sampling has the advantage of minimising bias, but "fixed" sampling has the virtue of operational convenience. In circumstances where there are multiple manufacturing conditions and in centres with large volumes of production, control testing should be increased above the statistically determined minimum to a level of approximately 1-10% of production in order to address process variations.

Whereas it is desirable to obtain the earliest possible indication of a non-conforming process, the number of samples that can be tested in any given period of time may be limited by practical considerations at the blood establishment. A basic goal is that the number of control samples tested in a pre-determined period should permit a statistically meaningful test of non-conformance in each period. Typically, this sample should be obtained over the course of one or two months of production, though adequate sampling over a briefer lapse of time is appropriate for the most safety-critical quality standards, and for centres that produce large volumes of products in relatively brief periods.

Two methods of statistical process control are provided below as examples.

EXAMPLE 1:

Method of scan statistics

The method of scan statistics provides one suitable model for determining the frequency of control testing. (See: Glaz, J., Naus, J., Wallenstein, S. Scan Statistics, New York 2001: Springer.) In this method, the number of non-conforming test results in a fixed sample size is determined. However, the sample set is regarded as a "window" of observations that "moves" progressively as test results are accumulated. For example, if the "window size" were set at 60 observations, the first test set would include observations one through 60. The second test set would include observations two through 61; the third test set would include observations three through 62; etc. (Progression of the "window" can also be done a few samples at a time, such as by addition of daily test results as a group.) To apply this method, the blood centre must identify a reasonably large "universe" of ultimate test samples, typically representing a year or more of testing, or a period after which routine re-validation might be expected to occur because of process modifications (e.g., equipment replacement, software upgrades, etc.) The size of the moving "window" can then be determined based on the expected rate of failed tests for a conforming process (as defined in the Quality Control Tables of each chapter), the size of the test "universe," and the "target rate" of failure to be detected as indicating a non-conforming process. Table 27 shows the minimum failure rate that can be detected at 80% or greater power in any single "window" of control tests for test criteria with false positive rates below 5%. Requiring that the number of control tests in the "window" should take place in the desired time interval yields the frequency of control testing.

The following example illustrates how the method of scan statistics can be used:

A blood centre seeks to monitor the failure rate of leukocyte reduction. The expected failure rate (rate of non-conforming tests for a conforming process) is taken to be 0.1%. The centre sets an action trigger at 5% as a means to detect a defective lot of filters. The quality control standard is set to assure, with at least 80% confidence, that a true failure rate of 5% would be detected, but at a false-positive rate below 5% for declaration of non-conformance.

For a blood centre with 400 QC tests per year (approximately 34 per month), a non-conforming process can be declared if in any "moving window" of 60 consecutive QC tests, 2 or more non-conforming test results are found (i.e. the "trigger" is greater than 1 non-conforming test in any window of 60 tests.). This model has a power of 80.8% to detect a true rate of non-conformance of 5% in any window of 60 tests, and near certainty to detect this rate over one year. Based on scan statistics, the false-positive rate of such declarations is only 2.0%.

If the number of QC tests is 1200 per year (100 per month), a non-conforming process can be declared if in any "moving window" of 120 sequential QC tests, 3 or more non-conforming test results are found. The false-positive rate of such declarations is only 0.7%. The power is 80.7% to detect a non-conformance rate of 4.6% (power is 85.6% to detect a 5% failure rate) for any window of 120 tests, and near certainty over one year.

Table 27: Sample Size ("Window") and Maximum Number of Failed Tests Allowed For A Conforming Process Based on Scan Statistics

Allowed Failure Rate for a Conforming Process	Number of Tests in "Universe" (e.g. the number of tests per year)	Sample Size (i.e. the Fixed Number of Tests in a moving "Window")	Maximum Allowed Number of Failed Tests in Window	False Positive Rate of Test Criterion	Minimum Failure Rate of a Non-conforming Process Detectable at >80% Power in Any Single "Window"	
					Minimum "Target rate" of Failure for a Non-Conforming Process	Power to Detect non-conforming Process in any window of QC tests
25%	400	30	16	2.5%	63%	81.9%
		60	26	2.9%	50%	81.7%
	1200	30	17	2.0%	66%	81.3%
		60	27	3.8%	52%	83.0%
10%	400	30	9	3.5%	40%	82.4%
		60	14	2.7%	30%	83.8%
	1200	30	10	2.8%	43%	81.1%
5%	400	30	6	3.7%	29%	81.0%
		60	9	2.3%	21%	83.7%
	1200	30	7	2.2%	33%	82.3%
1%	400	30	3	1.0%	18%	81.4%
		60	4	0.9%	11%	80.3%
	1200	60	4	2.7%	11%	80.3%
0.1%	400	30	1	1.1 %	10%	81.6%
		60	1	2.0%	5%	80.8%
	1200	30	1	3.2%	10%	81.6%
		120	2	0.7%	4.6%	80.7%

EXAMPLE 2

Use of control charts

By plotting historical and prospective data on specially constructed charts, signs of process change can often be detected at an early stage, enabling remedial action to be taken. Steps for the construction of SPC charts are the same for all applications:

- collection of historical data;
- calculation of "location and variation statistics" (see below);
- calculation of statistical control limits for the location and variation statistics;
- constructions of the chart;
- plotting of prospective data.

Two types of data are conventionally collected:

- variable data, appropriate to anything which is measured directly such as cell count, pH, time taken for a process, etc.;
- attribute data, appropriate to anything which is counted on a "yes or no" basis.

The type of SPC chart used depends on the type of data collected.

Control charts for variable data

The major applications in a blood centre are likely to be Individual/Moving Range charts, and Average/Range charts.

1) **Individual/Moving Range charts** are used where a process is monitored by a single measurement on the sample, of the parameter in question e.g. residual leukocyte count on a platelet preparation. The steps for constructing an SPC chart are as follows:

- historical data are collected by measuring a random sample each day, and the moving range established by taking the difference between each sample and its predecessor.
- the location statistic is the average of the individual counts; the variation statistic is the average moving range.
- the natural variation in a process has been defined as the process average plus or minus 3 standard deviations. Hence the Upper Control Limit (UCL) and Lower Control Limit (LCL) for the location statistic and variation statistics are determined as the appropriate average plus and minus 3 standard deviations.
- the SPC chart conventionally has two distinct parts: one for the location statistic which appears above the other for the variation statistic. For each, the average is drawn as a solid line between two dotted lines signifying the UCL and LCL.
- prospective data are plotted on the charts in a similar way.

2) **Average/Range charts** are used in a situation where an early statistical response to a small process change is required, and where multiple control samples (up to 10) are subjected to the process. A typical example might be the repeated use of a control sample during the daily use of a cytometer. In this situation, the average daily count on the control sample will be calculated, the location statistic being the average of the average. Each day will show a range in the control counts; the variation statistic is the average of these ranges. The Average/Range chart is then constructed in a similar manner to the Individual/Moving Range chart, except that the LCL for the Range part of the chart is, by definition, zero.

Control charts for attribute data

Attribute data will, in general, fall into one of two groups – those counting the number of units sampled which are defective, and those counting the incidence of non-conformance to a requirement, each non-conformance in this latter case being classified as a defect. For example, a completed form will be classified as defective if it contains even one non-conformance, even though it may in fact contain multiple defects.

1) **Attribute charts for proportion of defective units** (sometimes known as p-charts) are based on the calculation of the proportion of units found to be defective, i.e. one or more defects per unit sampled – in sets of units sampled at intervals. The location statistic for the attribute is calculated by dividing the total number of defectives by the total number of units sampled, unless the sets of samples are always the same size in which case the average of the proportion defective in each set may be taken. Since the data stem from yes/no criteria, attribute charts do not have a variation statistic.

    UCL and LCL are determined as before. In this system it is possible to arrive at a negative value for the LCL, in which case it defaults to zero.

    It should be noted that the calculation of standard deviation in a yes/no system such as this depends on the sample size, so that an increase or decrease in the set of units sampled will necessitate resetting of the UCL and LCL. An increase in sampling size will generally result in convergence of UCL and LCL, making the system more sensitive to change in the process.

    Construction of the chart is carried out as above.

2) **Attribute charts for defects** (sometimes known as u-charts) are generally useful when the object under investigation often has more than one non-conformance with requirements. They thus lend themselves well to the control of clerical procedures. Collection of historical data involves counting the number of defects in each unit of a set of samples, repeated at intervals.

    The location statistic is the average number of defects per unit, calculated by dividing the total number of defects in the total number of historical samples. As before, there is no variation statistic for attribute data.

    Once again, UCL and LCL is calculated on the basis of the location statistic plus and minus 3 standard deviations. Standard deviation in this system will again depend on sample size, and any prospective increase will require resetting of UCL and LCL.

    The likely result will be a convergence on the average, facilitating the detection of smaller changes in the process.

    Construction of the u-chart follows the convention set for all SPC charts.

Interpretation of control charts

In general, when plotting prospective data on the control chart follows the pattern established by the use of historical data in its construction, the process may be assumed to be "in control ". Changes in the pattern form a reliable and sensitive means of detecting that change has taken place in the process, warranting investigations into the cause. "Rules" have been established to give guidance to users as to when change has occurred, those usually employed being:

- Rule 1:   Any point outside one of the control limits

- Rule 2:   Seven consecutive points all above or all below the average line

- Rule 3:   Seven consecutive points all increasing or all decreasing (a particular indicator of drift in the process average or range)

In addition, any unusual pattern or trend within the control lines may be an indicator of change.

Should information from the charts indicate that unplanned change is taking place within the process, action should be taken to identify any specfic or common cause of the change. Application of SPC is the most reliable way of confirming that measures taken to improve the efficiency of a process are giving the desired results, by showing reduction in variation around the mean (for measured data) or a trend toward zero defects (for counted data).

PART E:
Transfusion practices

Chapter 28: Pre-transfusion measures

Prior to any transfusion of blood components, appropriate indications should be considered and documented.

1. Identification of patient at blood sampling

Samples for blood typing and compatibility testing must have a clear-cut identification. The following rules are recommended.

Patient identification shall be indicated on the tube label at the time of sampling. Family name and given name and birthdate will serve as a minimal requirement for identification. Normally it should be supplemented by a unique, new medical identification. In newborn infants, the sex and the number on the identification wrist band is noted in addition. If it is not possible to establish a patients' identity, a unique series of numbers may be used on wrist bands and attached to the patient according to specified rules.

The identification system should link the patient identification, the operator, the blood sample through processing and the blood product and should confirm the original patient identification at the time of blood administration. Emphasis must be placed on error recognition.

In immediate relation to sampling, the data on the tube label must be checked either by asking the patient to tell his/her name and birthdate, and/or by reading these or other data on a wrist band securely attached to the patient. This identity control shall be done even if the patient is known to the phlebotomist, who with his/her signature on the order form shall certify that it has been performed.

Blood samples which are inappropriately labelled should always be refused for blood typing and/or compatibility testing.

2. Blood group serological investigations

These include blood typing, antibody screening and compatibility testing before transfusion of red cell products.

a) Blood typing

The ABO and RhD blood type and, when needed, other blood types, shall be performed before transfusions except in emergencies when a delay may be life-threatening and typing may be carried out in parallel with transfusion of the blood components. It is further recommended that antibody screening for the detection of irregular erythrocyte antibodies be carried out in conjunction with patient blood typing.

The normal procedure shall be to make the investigation in due time before expected transfusions, e.g. in elective surgery.

The laboratory must have a reliable and validated procedure for blood typing which will include double-checking of data at the time of issuing a report on the blood group, and other serological findings, for inclusion in the patient's clinical record.

b) Compatibility testing

The compatibility between donor and recipient must be assured in transfusions of components containing amounts of red cells visible to the naked eye.

Ideally compatibility testing should be carried out on repeat samples other than the one used in initial blood typing but should, in any case, be carried out on a sample taken no more than 4 days before the proposed transfusion for patients who have not been transfused or pregnant during the last three months.

The basis for compatibility is a correctly determined ABO and RhD blood type in donor and recipient. When clinically significant erythrocyte antibodies are present in the patient's circulation, only red cells which lack the corresponding antigens should be selected for transfusion.

Compatibility testing between donor red cells and recipient's serum shall be done in all cases with irregular erythrocyte antibodies. It is recommended as a routine procedure even when no antibodies have been found but may be omitted if other measures (e.g. type and screen, see below) are taken to guarantee safety. The compatibility testing shall include a sufficiently reliable and validated technique to guarantee detection of irregular erythrocyte antibodies, such as the indirect antiglobulin technique.

A type and screen procedure, where used as a replacement for compatibility testing, must include:

1.   a reliable and validated, preferably by computer, checking procedure when the blood units are delivered;

2.   test cells which cover all antigens, preferably homozygous, corresponding to the vast majority of clinically important antibodies;

3.   sufficiently sensitive techniques for the detection of erythrocyte antibodies;

4.   laboratory records of tests performed and of the disposition of all units handled (including patient identification).

A sample of the serum used for cross-matching or antibody screening should be retained in a frozen state for a period of time determined by national regulations.

Chapter 29: Transfusion

1. Safety measures

The medical person who gives the transfusion to a patient is responsible for the control of identity and other safety measures.

Verification of identity shall be carried out both by asking the patient to tell his/her name and date of birth and by reading these or other identification details on a wrist-band which has been attached to the patient according to well-specified rules.

Verification that the relevant infusion operators are being used according to manufacturer's recommendations shall be carried out by a medical officer before attaching the blood components unit. It is recommended that no transfusion sets are used for more than 6 hours. Verification that there is no visible deterioration of the blood components shall be carried out with particular emphasis on discoloration.

Verification of compatibility between patient and blood unit shall be carried out by:

1. comparing the identity information received from the patient with data on the laboratory's certificate of compatibility testing (if appropriate);
2. checking the certificate of the patient's blood group against the blood group denoted on the blood unit label;
3. checking that the expiry date of the blood unit has not been passed;
4. recording the identity of the patient.

The identification number and nature of the units transfused shall be noted in the patient's record so that the donors can be traced if necessary.

2. Clinical surveillance

During transfusion of blood components careful observation of the patient is mandatory. This applies particularly in the first 15 minutes of the transfusion where significant transfusion reactions are more likely to occur and in the transfusion of any component prepared by an open system.

Blood components should be transfused within the recommended time to avoid compromising clinical effectiveness and safety.

3. Warming of blood

Rapid transfusion of cold blood may be dangerous. Any warming device used must be controlled and monitored to ensure that the correct temperature of the blood has been achieved.

4. Addition of medicinal products or infusion solutions to components

Because of the risk of damage to the blood components no medicinal products or infusion solutions may be added to blood units.

5. Handling of frozen units

Frozen units have to be handled with great care since the containers may be brittle and may easily crack at low temperatures.

If thawing in a water bath, steps should be taken to prevent contamination of the administration ports.

After thawing of frozen plasma the content shall be inspected to ensure that all cryoprecipitate has been dissolved and that the container is not damaged. Containers which leak must be discarded. Thawed preparations should be transfused as soon as possible (and must not be refrozen).

6. The risk of air embolism

During blood transfusion, air embolism is possible under some circumstances if the operator is not sufficiently careful and skilful.

7. Transfusion complications

Transfusion complications include adverse reactions and even failure of expected therapeutic response.

As each transfusion of blood components is a separate biological event, careful notation and reporting of any observed reaction is the responsibility of the attending physician (see paragraph on "side-effects" under each specific chapter).

It is also important to determine the efficacy of the transfusion of the specific component by recording appropriate pre- and post-transfusion parameters.

Complications may occur, either in direct relation to the transfusion or with a delay of hours or days. All serious complications shall be investigated, mild reactions according to the judgment of the responsible physician.

When a serious complication after transfusion of red cell preparations has occurred and the patient shows chills, fever, breathing difficulties, shock, or hypotension, back pain (which cannot be related to the patient's underlying disease) the following shall be investigated.

a. Check all identification of recipient and blood product.

b. Check that the ABO and RhD blood group of the blood unit label is compatible with the patient's blood group certificate. If irregular antibodies outside the ABO and RhD systems are present, check if blood of compatible blood type has been used.

c. A blood sample taken before the transfusion (may be available at the compatibility testing laboratory); a blood sample taken after the transfusion, the blood unit with the transfusion set maintained in site, and the pilot tube shall be sent for investigation. It is recommended that this include a direct smear and a bacterial culture test of the content of the blood unit, a serological investigation for blood group incompatibility, and inspection of the blood unit for any damage.

In the case of repeated, febrile non-haemolytic transfusion reactions, the use of leukocyte-poor blood for subsequent transfusions is recommended. If it happens for prevention of febrile non-haemolytic reaction associated with platelets transfusion, non steroid anti-inflammatory drugs should be used.

Long-term complications may occur. These include mainly alloimmunisation and disease transmission. As this text is not intended to be comprehensive in this area readers are advised to consult appropriate publications.

There should be co-operation between the physician and the blood banks to facilitate investigations of possible transfusion transmitted infections and to provide medical follow up of recipient in cases where a donor is subsequently found to have seroconverted.

Appropriate follow up and patient counselling is also necessary when significant alloimmunisation against transfused cells may have taken place (see Chapter 30).

8. Hospital transfusion committees

Establishment of hospital transfusion committees is to be encouraged.

A hospital blood transfusion committee should include representatives of the blood establishment and the main clinical units with a significant transfusion activity. It is recommended that physicians, nurses and administrative personnel be represented.

The main goals of a hospital blood transfusion committee are:

- to define blood transfusion policies adapted to the local clinical activities;
- to conduct regular evaluation of blood transfusion practices;
- to analyse any undesirable events due to blood transfusion;
- to take any corrective measures if necessary;
- to ensure that all staff involved in transfusion practice receive adequate training.

Similarly, systems of audit of the clinical use of components will further enhance the efficacy of transfusion practice.

Chapter 30: Haemovigilance

1. Definition

Haemovigilance is defined as the organised surveillance procedures related to serious adverse or unexpected events or reactions in donors or recipients and the epidemiological follow up of donors.

The ultimate goal of haemovigilance is to prevent the recurrence of adverse events and reactions. For that purpose, the results of data analysis should be fed back periodically to their providers and communicated to any competent authority, indicating, whenever possible, any preventive or corrective measure to be adopted.

Haemovigilance should also incorporate an early alert/warning system.

The information provided by haemovigilance may contribute to improving the safety of blood collection and transfusion by:

- providing the medical community with a reliable source of information about adverse events and reactions associated with blood collection and transfusion;

- indicating corrective measures required to prevent the recurrence of some incidents or dysfunctions in the transfusion process;

- warning hospitals and blood establishments about adverse events and reactions that could involve more individuals than a single recipient, including:

  - those related to the transmission of infectious diseases;
  - those related to blood bags, solutions or blood processing.

2. Prerequisites for implementation of a haemovigilance network

Haemovigilance should be a responsibility of the competent national authority for blood safety. Haemovigilance networks should embody operational linkages between clinical departments, hospital blood banks, blood establishments, and national authorities.

3. Traceability of blood components

Traceability, which is a prerequisite for haemovigilance, may be defined as the ability to trace each individual unit of blood or blood components derived thereof from the donor to its final destination, whether this is a patient, a manufacturer of medicinal products or disposal, and vice versa.

Traceability can provide information on the total number of:

- patients that have been transfused;

- blood units or components that have been used;

- blood donors that have provided the transfused blood units or components.

Without this information, it is difficult to calculate the incidence of adverse events and reactions and thus to estimate risk. The number of adverse events and reactions, over a given time period, may help in identifying critical issues within the process.

Traceability should cover also cases in which the blood unit or component is not transfused to a patient, but is used for the manufacturing of medicinal products or for research and investigational purposes, or disposed of.

The essential element for traceability is a unique identification numeric or alphanumeric code for each donation, with a subsidiary code for each component prepared from that donation*. This unique identifier must be linked with data identifying both the donor and the recipient, so that all patients transfused with a particular donor's blood or all donors who donated the blood components a patient received may be traced.

By this system the following data should be made unmistakeably available:

a. personal data uniquely identifying the donor and providing a means to contact him/her;

b. the blood establishment in which blood or blood component collection has been carried out;

c. the date of donation;

d. the blood components produced and additional component information, if appropriate;

---

* Documentation and record-keeping to guarantee the traceability of blood and blood products especially in hospital" Recommendation N°R (96) 11 of the Council of Europe.

e. the blood establishment or hospital blood bank to which the blood component has been distributed, if different from the production facility;

f. the hospital and the ward to which the blood component has been issued for transfusion;

g. the date and time of issue;

h. the final fate of the unit; either the identity of the patient who received it or other use (e.g. quality assurance, reagents, discards, etc.);

i. the date and starting time of transfusion.

In case of blood components that have not been issued for transfusion, data should be available to identify the facility where the units have been used or disposed of.

Information systems should be available to facilitate rapid traceability by using patients, blood components and donors as data-access keys. To ensure the reliability of the data base, confirmation that the blood component was transfused to the patient for whom it was issued is needed. Without this, proving the link between donor and patient would require verification in the patient's notes that the blood component had been transfused. The document confirming the transfusion should also include information on the existence or non existence of immediate adverse events or reactions.

4. Co-operation between blood establishments, hospital blood banks and clinical departments

Reporting and analysis of adverse events and reactions associated with transfusion requires close co-operation between the clinical department where transfusion took place, the hospital blood bank that issued the transfused blood component and the blood establishment that collected and distributed the blood unit, if different from the hospital blood bank. This co-operation is essential to ensure a complete investigation of any adverse event or reaction including uneventful transfusion errors. In the blood establishment and/or in the hospital blood bank, the physician involved may be the one responsible for blood component delivery, or a physician specifically in charge of haemovigilance. Similarly, in the clinical departments, the involved person can be the physician in charge of the patient, or another physician specifically in charge of haemovigilance.

It should be stressed that the responsibility of reporting adverse events and reactions does not imply the responsibility for individual patient's care.

5. Standardisation of reporting

Reports of adverse events and reactions should be made in the same way in all the institutions that participate in the haemovigilance network. This implies not only the use of common report forms, but also a common training programme ensuring among all participants a similar way of interpretation for a given incident, and a common and agreed definition of the different types of adverse events and reactions. In this respect, the persons specifically in charge of haemovigilance may contribute to the standardisation both of reports and of definitions.

In practice, to be achieved, standardisation of reporting requires an active training policy initiated inside the network.

6. Data analysis

All the reports should be carefully analysed before inclusion in the haemovigilance data base which can be exploited at different levels: institutional, regional, national or international. Whatever the magnitude of the network, an individual institution should have permanent access to its own data.

7. Type of adverse events and reactions collected in the haemovigilance network

7.1 Adverse reactions in patients

Adverse reactions associated with transfusion of blood components are the primary scope of a haemovigilance system, which should collect reports concerning patients of events such as:

- immediate reactions during transfusion, such as haemolysis, non haemolytic febrile transfusion reaction, rash, erythema, urticaria, anaphylactic shock, bacterial contamination, TRALI, etc.;

- delayed untoward effects after transfusion, such as haemolysis, acute GvHD, post-transfusion purpura, ALT increase, haemochromatosis, etc.;

- virus transmission;

- occurrence of alloimmunisation against red cell, HLA or platelet antigens.

The rules for reporting may differ according to the type and severity of adverse reaction. In case of minor reactions such as non haemolytic febrile transfusion reaction, rash, erythema and urticaria, individual reports should be sent only by the clinical departments to the blood bank, which, depending on the organisation of the haemovigilance network, may send periodic reports to its blood establishment or to the competent authority concerning the incidence of such events.

On the contrary, in case of serious adverse reactions in blood recipients, which may be related to the transfused blood components, notification should be sent as soon as possible to the blood establishment where the components have been collected.

Prompt reporting enables the blood establishment to take action to block blood components from related donors, donations or production methods. This applies to any event that may involve several individuals, and to serious hazards. Moreover, in case of viral transmission the extent of required investigations should be clearly defined.

Serious adverse reactions include: acute haemolytic transfusion reaction, sepsis due to bacterial contamination, delayed haemolysis, transfusion related acute lung injury, transfusion associated graft versus host disease, transfusion transmitted viral infections, anaphylaxis, transfusion associated circulatory overload.

7.2   *Adverse reactions in donors*

Haemovigilance deals also with donors and blood donation, and should gather information on:

- adverse reactions observed during blood donation;

- data related to donor selection, such as frequency and causes of blood donation exclusion;

- epidemiologic data on the donors found confirmed positive in infectious marker screening.

These data, collected within the blood establishments, should be reported at least annually to the national haemovigilance system and/or to the competent authority. Particular attention should be given to serious adverse reactions such as syncope with trauma, cardiac failure, nerve, arterial damage or infection at venipuncture site.

7.3   *Adverse events*

Adverse events are defined as any untoward occurrence associated with the collecting, testing, processing, storage and distribution of blood and blood components that might lead to an adverse reaction in blood recipients or blood donors.

Serious adverse events are those which might lead to death or life-threatening, disabling or incapacitating conditions for patients or donors, or which results in or prolongs hospitalisation or morbidity. Examples of these serious adverse events are failures to detect an infectious agent, errors in ABO typing, wrong labelling of blood components or blood samples. As of Directive EC 2002/98, these events are to be notified.

"Near-miss" events are a subgroup of adverse events, defined as any error, which if undetected, could result in the determination of a wrong blood group or undetection of a red cell antibody, or issue, collection, or administration of an incorrect, inappropriate or unsuitable component, but which was recognised before transfusion took place.

Uneventful transfusion errors are another subgroup of adverse events defined as any incorrect, inappropriate or unsuitable component transfusion which causes no harm to the recipient. For example, administration of a mismatched ABO compatible component or failure to give irradiated components when prescribed.

Near misses and uneventful transfusion errors notification may contribute in identifying systematic inadequacies in the safety procedures adopted for the clinical transfusion process, before any serious hazard occurs. Therefore, the haemovigilance system should provide to all the staff, both of blood establishments and hospital blood banks and of the clinical departments, adequate information on the importance of this kind of events and facilitate their reporting through anonymous forms, in order to avoid any blame on the involved personnel. The haemovigilance system should also foster the implementation of information technology, such as barcodes and barcode readers, in the critical steps of the process, such as the identification of blood donors, donor samples and donated units, and of patients, of blood samples drawn for pre-transfusion testing and of blood components issued for transfusion to an assigned recipient.

8. Tracing and retrieval of potentially infectious donations (HIV, HCV or HBV)

8.1. *Post-transfusion infection reported to the blood establishment*

Hospitals should inform the blood establishment whenever a recipient of blood products develops laboratory tests results and/or disease symptoms, indicating that a blood product may have been infectious for hepatitis (B or C) or HIV. It is important that the blood establishment is informed by the hospital, so to allow further action on implicated donations and donors, in order to prevent harm to other recipients.

The blood establishment should request relevant information from the hospital or the general physician about the infection and the recipient's course of disease and possible risk factors in the recipient for the infection.

Where feasible and appropriate, the blood establishment should (temporarily) defer all implicated donors from further donations, and retrieve (temporarily) or quarantine all in-date components for transfusion collected from the implicated donors.

The blood establishment should establish a plan of investigation, the results of which should be recorded. Test results from donations of the implicated donors may be re-analysed, or additional or confirmatory tests on archived samples or freshly obtained samples from the implicated donors may be performed with the aim to exclude HIV, HCV or HBV infection in the donor(s). If such analysis reasonably excludes infection, such donor(s) may be re-released for future donations, and (temporarily) blocked products derived from their donations may be re-released.

Whenever an implicated donor is found with a confirmed positive test for HIV, HCV or HBV infection, the blood establishment should act accordingly with regard to deferral of the donor and look-back procedure on previous potentially infectious donations and inform the hospital concerned.

The incident is reported to the national haemovigilance system and/or competent authorities.

8.2. *Post donation information*

Blood donors should be instructed to inform the blood establishment when signs or symptoms occur after a donation, indicating that the donation may have been infectious. A donor may also inform the blood establishment that he or she previously donated blood, but should not have done so in the light of donor selection criteria aimed at the health protection of recipients, e.g.: in retrospect did not fulfil criteria mentioned in the donor questionnaire.

The blood establishment should (temporarily) block all in-house products from the donor and retrieve all in-date products. The relevant plasma fractionation institute must be notified.

The blood establishment should perform a risk analysis to assess whether the incident indicates a potentially infectious blood product for recipient(s). Test results from donations of the implicated donors may be re-analysed, or additional or confirmatory tests on archived samples or freshly obtained samples from the donor may be performed.

In case a confirmed HBV, HCV or HIV infection is shown in the donor, the blood establishment should act accordingly with regard to deferral of the donor and lookback procedure on previous potentially infectious donations.

8.3. Retrieval of blood products

The blood establishment retrieves in date blood products from the hospital(s) as a precautionary measure in case of a quality deviation. This may be a temporary measure and implies that certain retrieved blood products may be re-released after proper risk analysis and/or additional testing. The measure is taken in order to prevent harm to potential recipients.

8.4. Tracing of recipients of potentially infectious blood (lookback)

The blood establishment initiates a lookback procedure which is aimed at the tracing of recipients of blood components from a potentially infectious blood donation and notification of these recipient(s) by their treating physicians, whenever a blood donation may have taken place within the window period of a (repeat) donor with a confirmed HIV, HBV or HCV infection. Implicated donations include those within a time frame equal to the maximum test specific window period of the infection, preceding a negative screening test result in the donor.

The blood establishment should inform the hospital in writing about the incident and advise the hospital to trace the recipient(s) of the implicated blood product(s) and inform the treating physician about the potentially infectious transfusion.

It is the responsibility of the treating physician to inform the recipient about the potentially infectious transfusion, unless there are medical arguments not to do so. If the recipient is tested, in order to establish or to exclude the infection, the blood establishment should be informed by the hospital about such test results. If testing of the recipient is not performed, the blood establishment should also be informed of this by the hospital.

If the recipient is confirmed to be positive for the infection the incident is reported to a national haemovigilance system and / or competent authorities.

Consistent with the recommendations of the competent public health authority, blood establishments should consider the need to trace and notify blood component recipients and/or their physicians in cases where a blood donor subsequently is diagnosed with vCJD infection, and the means of doing this.

8.5. Contract between the blood establishment and the hospital

In those situations in which blood collection and processing is carried out in facilities located outside the hospitals, the above procedures may be described in the contract(s) between the blood establishment and the hospital(s).

9. Minimum information to be captured

Information about transfused patients must be managed according to the country's confidentiality requirements.

9.1. Patients information

Identification should include at least date of birth, sex, and unique patient number. Clinical signs observed should be documented, in a standardised fashion, either specific for a given adverse event or reaction, or the same form for every untoward effect. Clinical outcome of an adverse reaction should be stated.

9.2. Component information

This information should include a detailed prescription of the component involved:

- unit number and adequate codes for components and donor identification;
- description of the component, including:
- the type of component, i.e. red cell, platelet or plasma;
- the type of preparation, i.e. from whole blood or from apheresis;
- other characteristics, i.e. leukodepleted, irradiated, plasma reduced, etc.;
- conditions and duration of storage prior to transfusion.

9.3. Information about severity

Severity should be graded. A suggested scale may be:

- (0): no sign;
- (1): immediate signs without vital risk and full resolution;
- (2): immediate signs with vital risk;
- (3): long term morbidity;
- (4): death of the patient.

9.4. Imputability

The possible relationship between the observed adverse reaction and the blood components given should be identified. A suggested scale may be:

Imputability scale		Explanation
0	Excluded	When there is conclusive evidence beyond reasonable doubts for attributing the adverse reaction to alternative causes.
0	Unlikely	When the evidence is clearly in favour of attributing the adverse reaction to causes other than the blood or blood components.
NA	Not assessable	When there is insufficient data for causality assessment.
1	Possible	When the evidence is indeterminate for attributing adverse reaction either to the blood or blood component or to alternative causes.
2	Likely, Probable	When the evidence is clearly in favour of attributing the adverse reaction to the blood or blood component.
3	Certain	When there is conclusive evidence beyond reasonable doubt for attributing the adverse reaction to the blood or blood component.

9.5. Information about the type of event

Report forms should enable differentiation between adverse events and reactions in patients and donors, near misses and uneventful transfusion errors.

9.6. *Summary*

Report forms should include a brief summary describing the event as well as the corrective actions taken.

9.7. *Other useful information*

a. In order to provide an evaluation of the incidence of untoward effects, each participating institution should provide the number of blood components used per year and the number of patients transfused, together with details of all reported events.

b. Additional information about the current guidelines and procedures in regard to the use of blood components will be useful in comparison of results from different institutions or even different countries.

10. Conclusion

Haemovigilance provides useful information on the morbidity of blood donation and transfusion, and gives guidance on corrective measures to prevent the recurrence of some incidents.

Moreover, haemovigilance must be considered as a part of total health care vigilance, along with pharmacovigilance, and vigilance on medical devices.

Acknowledgements

In 1988, the Select Committee on Quality Assurance in Blood Transfusion Services was requested by the Committee of Experts on Blood Transfusion and Immunohaematology to prepare the work hereafter on the basis of the 1986 publication on Quality Control in Blood Transfusion Services as well as of experience and practice of the laboratories and blood transfusion services represented on the committee.

In 2005, the following members of the Select Committee of Experts drafted this 12th edition:

Prof Dr Dieter SCHÖNITZER
Head of Zentralinstitut für Bluttransfusion und Immunologische Abteilung, Landeskrankenhaus, Universitätsklinik Innsbruck
Anichstrasse 35, A-6020 Innsbruck (AUSTRIA)
E-mail : Diether.Schoenitzer@tilak.or.at

Prof Dr Danielle SONDAG-THULL
Director, Blood Transfusion Service of the Red Cross (French part)
41, rue Dos Fanchon B-4020 Liege (BELGIUM)
E-mail: d.sondag@redcross.be

Dr Svetla BAKALOVA, Ass. Prof, PhD
Department Quality Assurance, National Centre for Haematology and Transfusiology
Plovdivsko pole str. 6. Sofia 1759 (BULGARIA)
E-mail: bakalovasvetla@abv.bg / ncht-bg@abv.bg

Dr Morten BAGGE HANSEN, MD DMSc
Blood establishment, Section 2034
Rigshospitalet, Blegdamsvej 9, DK-2100 Copenhagen (DENMARK)
E-mail : bagge@dadlnet.dk

Dr Tom KRUSIUS, MD, PhD
Medical Director, Finnish Red Cross Blood Transfusion service
Kivihaantie 7, FIN - 00310 Helsinki 31 (FINLAND)
E-mail: tom.krusius@bts.redcross.fi / seija.saana@stm.fi

Dr Georges ANDREU
Etablissement Français du Sang
100, avenue de Suffren F-75015 Paris (FRANCE)
E-mail : georges.andreu@efs.sante.fr

Prof. Dr med Harald KLÜTER
Institut für Transfusionsmedizin und Immunologie Fakultät für Klinische
Medizin Mannheim der Universität Heidelberg
Friedrich-Ebert-Strasse 107 D- 68167 Mannheim (GERMANY)
E-mail: h.klueter@blutspende.de

Prof. Dr György MEDGYESI
Scientific adviser Headquarters Hungarian National Blood Transfusion
Service
19-21 Karolina ut Budapest - XI mailing address: H-1518 Budapest, P.O. Box
44 (HUNGARY)
E-mail: medgyesi.gyorgy@ogyi.hu

Dr Sveinn GUDMUNDSSON
Director Blood Bank
University Hospital IS-101 Reikjavik (ICELAND)
E-mail: sveinn@landspitali.is

Dr Joan O'RIORDAN
Irish Blood Transfusion Service, National Blood Centre
St James Street, IR-Dublin 8 (IRELAND)
E-mail: joriordan@ibts.ie

Dr Maurizio MARCONI
Centro Trasfusionale e di Immunologia dei Trapianti, IRCCS
Ospedale Maggiore, Via F. Sforza 35, 20122 Milano (ITALY)
E-mail : mmarconi@policlinico.mi.it

Dr Cees L. van der POEL
Secretary Medical Affairs, Stichting Sanquin
Bloedvoorziening, P.O. Box 9892, NL-1066 AN Amsterdam (NETHERLANDS)
E-mail: c.vanderpoel@sanquin.nl

Prof Dr Bjarte SOLHEIM
IMMI Rikshospitalet
N-0027 Oslo (NORWAY)
E-mail: bjarte.solheim@rikshospitalet.no

Dr Magdalena LETOWSKA
Institute of Haematology and Blood Transfusion
ul. Chocimska 5, PL-00957 Warsaw (POLAND)
E-mail: letowska@ihit.waw.pl

Dr Fatima NASCIMENTO
Servico de Imuno-Hemoterapia Hospital de Santa Maria
Av. Professor Egas Moniz , Lisboa (PORTUGAL)
E-mail: fatima.nascimento@hsm.min-saude.pt

Dr Nada VASILJEVIC
National Co-ordinator of the National Blood Transfusion Project for Serbia
Lamartinova 21 11000 Belgrade (SERBIA AND MONTENEGRO)
E-mail: nada99@eunet.yu / gusic@eunet.yu

Dr Zoran STANOJKOVIC
Blood Transfusion Centre
Bulevar dr. Zorana Djindjica 48 18000 Nis (SERBIA AND MONTENEGRO)
E-mail: ztknis@bankerinter.net

Dra. Maria PAZ MARTIN HERNANDEZ
Hospital La Mancha, Centro Servicio de Hematologia
Avda. De la Constitución No. 3 E-13600 Alcázar de San Juan, Ciudad Real
(SPAIN)
E-mail: mpmartin@msc.es

Dr Jan SÄFWENBERG -Dept. of Clinical Immunology and Transfusion Medicine
University Hospital, SE-75185 Uppsala (SWEDEN)
E-mail: jan.safwenberg@clm.uas.lul.se

Prof. Manuel FREY-WETTSTEIN -Zürcher Blutspendedienst SRK
Hirschengraben 60, CH-8001 Zürich (SWITZERLAND)
E-mail : m.frey-wettstein@zhbsd.ch

Dr Brian McCLELLAND
Scottish National Blood Transfusion Service
Ellen's Glen Road, Edinburgh EH17 7QT (UNITED KINGDOM)
E-mail: Brian.McClelland@snbts.csa.scot.nhs.uk

Dr Jay S. EPSTEIN
Director, Office of Blood Research and Review, Center for Biologics,
Evaluation and Research
Food and Drug Administration (FDA), HFM-300, 1401 Rockville Pike, Rockville,
MD 20852-1448, (USA)
E-mail: epsteinj@al.cber.fda.gov

Dr Peter FLANAGAN
National Medical Director, New Zealand Blood Service, National Office
71, Great South Road, PO Box 26611, NZ-EPSOM, Auckland (NEW ZEALAND)
E-mail: peter.flanagan@nzblood.co.nz

Dr Peter R. GANZ
Director Centre for Biologics Evaluation Biologic and Genetic Therapies
Directorate Health
Canada Building NO.6, Room 3364, AL 0603C3 Tunney's Pasture Ottawa,
Ontario K1A 0L2 (CANADA)
E-mail: peter_ganz@hc-sc.gc.ca

Dr Richard PEMBREY
Clinical Adviser, Blood and Tissues Unit, Office of Devices
Blood and Tissues Therapeutic Goods Administration (TGA)
Postal address: PO Box 100, Woden, ACT, 2606, (AUSTRALIA)
Street address: 136, Narrabundah Lanen, Sysmonston, ACT, 2609,
(AUSTRALIA)
E-mail: richard.pembrey@health.gov.au

Dr Tony KELLER
National Donor and Product Safety Manager
International Federation of Red Cross and Red Crescent Societies
97 Great Eastern Highway Rivervale WA 6103
Postal: GPO Box B80 Perth WA 6840 (AUSTRALIA)
E-mail: Akeller@arcbs.redcross.org.au

CO-ORDINATION

Karl-Friedrich BOPP
Head of Health Division, Council of Europe,
F-67075 Strasbourg Cedex. (FRANCE)
Tel: 33 3 88 41 22 14 / Fax: 33 3 88 41 27 26
E-mail: karl-friedrich.bopp@coe.int

Jacqueline LOSTAO
Administrator, Health Division, Council of Europe,
F-67075 Strasbourg Cedex. (FRANCE)
Tel: 33 3 88 41 2847 / Fax: 33 3 88 41 27 26
E-mail: jacqueline.lostao@coe.int

Susie MORGAN-CUNY
Administrative assistant, Health Division, Council of Europe,
F-67075 Strasbourg Cedex. (FRANCE)
Tel: 33 3 88 41 35 48 / Fax: 33 3 88 41 27 26
E-mail: susie.morgan@coe.int

Caroline HILLER
Assistant, Health Division, Council of Europe,
F-67075 Strasbourg Cedex (FRANCE)
Tel: 33.3.88.41.21.53 / Fax: 33 3 88 41 27 26
E-mail: caroline.hiller@coe.int

Health Department Web Site:
http://www.coe.int/T/E/Social_Cohesion/Health

Appendix 1: List of definitions

Additive solution	Solution specifically formulated to maintain beneficial properties of cellular components during storage
Adverse event	Any untoward occurrence associated with the collecting, testing, processing, storage and distribution of blood and blood components that might lead to an adverse reaction in blood recipients or blood donors
Adverse reaction	Unintended response in donor or in patient associated with the collection or transfusion of blood or blood components
Allogeneic donation	Blood and blood components collected from an individual and intended for transfusion to another individual, for use in medical devices or as source material for manufacturing into medicinal products.
Antibody quantitation	Technique routinely used to measure the level of antibody, i.e. anti-D (or anti-c) antibody in maternal sera.
Antiglobulin testing technique	The direct antiglobulin test (direct Coombs' test) detects antibody or complement bound to erythrocytes in vivo.
Anti-IgA antibodies	IgG or occasionally IgM anti-IgA produced by a IgA-deficient patient. Severe anaphylactoid transfusion reactions can occur in such patients.

Apheresis

Method of obtaining one or more blood components by machine processing of whole blood in which the residual components of the blood are returned to the donor during or at the end of the process.

Audit programme

A systematic and independent examination to determine whether quality activities and related results comply with planned arrangements and whether these arrangements are implemented effectively and are suitable to achieve objectives.

Autologous donation

Blood and blood components collected from an individual, intended solely for subsequent autologous transfusion to the individual

Autologous donors

Individuals may donate blood for their own use if the need for blood can be anticipated and a donation plan developed

Autologous transfusion

Transfusion, in which the donor and the recipient are the same person and in which predeposited blood and blood components are used.

Blood

Whole Blood collected from a single donor and processed either for transfusion or further manufacturing.

Blood bag

Blood component unit

Blood component

Therapeutic components of blood (red cells, white cells, platelets, plasma) that can be prepared by centrifugation, filtration, and freezing using conventional blood bank methodology.

Blood component release

Process which enables a blood component to be released from a quarantine status by the use of systems and procedures to ensure that the finished product meets its release specifications.

Blood establishment	Any structure or body that is responsible for any aspect of the collection and testing of human blood or blood components, whatever their intended purpose, and their processing, storage and distribution when intended for transfusion. This does not include hospital blood banks.
Blood product	Any therapeutic product derived from human blood or plasma
Buffy coat	Blood component prepared by centrifugation of a unit of whole blood which contains a considerable proportion of the leukocytes and platelets.
Buoyant density centrifugation	Technique applicable for separation based on density differences between cells.
Cell free plasma	Plasma obtained by cross-flow filtration, when blood flows along a membrane with a pore size allowing free passage of plasma proteins but not of blood cells.
Cell separator	An instrument for apheresis
Counter current centrifugation (elutriation)	Technique where cells subjected simultaneously to a liquid flow and a centrifugal force in opposite directions tend to be separated according to their size.
CPD-Adenine (CDPA)	Citrate-Phosphate-Dextrose with Adenine is a preservative-anticoagulant solution used for whole blood collection.
Cryoprecipitate	Plasma component prepared from fresh frozen plasma by freeze-thaw precipitation of proteins and subsequent concentration and resuspension of the precipitated proteins in a small volume of the plasma.

Cryoprecipitate-depleted plasma	A component prepared from plasma by removal of cryoprecipitate
Cryopreservation	Prolongation of the storage life of blood components by freezing.
Cryopreserved platelets	A component prepared by the freezing of platelets and stored.
Cytapheresis	An apheresis procedure intended for the collection of a cellular component of blood, such as red cells, leukocytes or platelets.
Deferral	Suspension of the eligibility of an individual to donate blood or blood components, such suspension being either permanent or temporary.
Depth and surface filtration	Technique of filtration using a filter bed of fibres: owing to the specific properties of platelets and granulocytes as well as the low flexibility of lymphocytes, these cells are more easily trapped in such a filter than are red cells.
Distribution	Act of delivery of blood and blood components to other blood establishments, hospital blood banks and manufacturers of blood and plasma derived products. It does not include the issuing of blood or blood components for transfusion.
DMSO	Acronym: Dimethylsulfoxide used as a cell-cryoprotective agent for the storage of platelets and stem cells in the frozen state.
Donor	A person in normal health with a good medical history who voluntarily gives blood or plasma for therapeutic use.
Febrile transfusion reactions	A febrile response associated with the administration of blood.

First time donor	Someone who has never donated either blood or plasma.
Fresh frozen plasma	A component prepared from whole blood or from plasma collected by apheresis frozen to a temperature that will maintain the labile coagulation factors in a functional state.
G-CSF	Acronym: Granulocyte-colony-stimulating factor
Glycerol	Propanetriol, used as a cell-cryoprotective agent for the storage of red cells in the frozen state.
Granulocytes	A component consisting primarily of granulocytes suspended in plasma, obtained by single-donor apheresis.
Haematocrit	Result obtained by the measurement of the volume of red cells in blood, after centrifugation, expressed as a percentage or as a ratio in the SI system
Haematopoietic progenitor cells	HPC are primitive pluripotent cells capable of self renewal as well as differentiation and maturation into all haematopoietic lineages. They are found in bone marrow (bone marrow cells (BMC)), in the mononuclear cells of circulating blood (peripheral blood stem cells (PBSC)) and in umbilical cord blood (umbilical stem cells (USC)).
Haemovigilance	Organised surveillance procedures related to serious adverse or unexpected events or reactions in donors or recipients, and the epidemiological follow up of donors.
Hospital blood bank	Hospital unit which stores and distributes and may perform compatibility tests on blood and blood components exclusively for use within the hospital facilities including hospital based transfusion activities.

Inspection	Formal and objective control according to adopted standards to assess compliance with a given directive and other relevant legislation and to identify problems.
Leukocyte depletion	The removal of leukocytes from blood.
Peripheral blood stem cells (PBSC)	Primitive pluripotent cells capable of self renewal as well as differentiation and maturation into all haematopoietic lineages, and found in the mononuclear cells of circulating blood, (see haematopoietic progenitor cells).
Plasma	The liquid portion of anticoagulated blood remaining after separation from the cellular components.
Platelets, recovered	A component derived from fresh whole blood which contains the majority of the original platelet content.
Red cell apheresis	Red cell from an apheresis red cell donation.
Red cells	A component obtained from a single whole blood donation by removal of part of the plasma, without further processing.
Red cells, buffy coat removed (Red cells: BCR)	A component prepared from a single whole blood donation by the separation of part of the plasma and the buffy-coat layer from the red cells.
Red cells, cryopreserved	Red cells of a single whole blood donation with most of the plasma removed, deep frozen using a cryoprotectant solution.
Red cells, in additive solution (Red cells: AS)	A component prepared from a single whole blood donation by separation of part of the plasma with subsequent suspension of the red cells in appropriate nutrient solution.

Red cells, in additive solution, buffy coat removed (Red cells: AS-BCR)	A component prepared from a single whole blood donation by separation of part of the plasma and buffy-coat, and with subsequent resuspension of the red cells in an appropriate nutrient solution.
Red cells, leukocyte-depleted	A component obtained by removing the majority of leukocytes from red cells.
Regular donor	Someone who routinely donates their blood or plasma (i.e. within the last two years), in accordance with minimum time intervals, in the same donation centre.
Repeat donor	Someone who has donated before but not within the last two years in the same donation centre.
Rh Immune-globulin	Rh immune globulin specific for D is given routinely to Rh-negative mothers bearing Rh-positive infants to protect them from red cell exposure during pregnancy and delivery, and so prevent alloimmunisation
Serious adverse event	Any untoward occurrence associated with the collecting, testing, processing, storage and distribution of blood and blood components that might lead to death or life-threatening, disabling or incapacitating conditions for patients or which results in, or prolongs, hospitalisation or morbidity.
Serious adverse reaction	Unintended response in donor or in patient associated with the collection or transfusion of blood or blood components that is fatal, life-threatening, disabling, incapacitating, or which results in, or prolongs hospitalisation or morbidity.

Standard operating procedures (SOPs)	Detailed documents: (1) covering all Good Manufacturing Practice-compliant activities; (2) containing specifications where appropriate; (3) process/procedure based; (4) modular, and (5) reflecting current practice. They must be updated as appropriate, and new techniques must be evaluated and validated before being introduced, to ensure conformation with quality criteria.
Statistical process control	Method of quality control of a product or a process that relies on a system of analysis of an adequate sample size without the need to measure every product of the process.
Thrombopoietin	A cytokine that regulates specifically the megakaryocytic lineage.
Thrombotic thrombocytopenic purpura (TTP)	First described by MOSCHOWITZ this syndrome associates the classical pentad of clinical findings: (1) fever; (2) thrombocytopenia; (3) microangiopathic haemolytic anaemia; (4) neurological abnormalities, and (5) renal involvement.
Validation	Establishment of documented and objective evidence that the particular requirements for a specific intended use can be consistently fulfilled.
Washed red cells	A component derived from whole blood by centrifugation and removal of plasma, with subsequent washing of the red cells in an isotonic solution.
Whole blood	Single unprocessed blood donation.
Xenotransplantation	Xenotransplantation is defined as any procedure that involves the transplantation or infusion into a human recipient of live animal cells, tissues or organs, or human body fluids, cells, tissues or organs that have ex vivo contact with live animal cells, tissues or organs.

Appendix 2: Principal abbreviations

AIDS = *Acquired Immune Deficiency Syndrome*

ALT = *Alanine Amino Transferase*

AS = *Additive Solution*

AS-BCR = *Additive Solution-Buffy Coat Removed*

BCR = *Buffy Coat Removed*

BPAT = *Batch Pre-Acceptance Testing*

BSA = *Bovine Serum Albumin*

CJD = *Creutzfeldt-Jacob Disease*

CMV = *CytoMegaloVirus*

GMP = *Good Manufacturing Practice*

GCSF = *Granulocyte Colony Stimulating Factor*

GVHD = Graft-Versus-Host Disease

Hb = *Haemoglobin*

HBcAb = *Hepatitis B core Antibody*

HBsAg = *Hepatitis B surface Antigen*

Hct = *Haematocrit*

HCV = *Hepatitis C Virus*

HLA = *Human Leukocyte Antigen*

HPA = *Human Platelet Antigen*

HPCs = *Haematopoietic Progenitor Cells*

HIV = *Human Immunodeficiency Virus*

HTLV = *Human T Leukaemia Virus*

LISS = *Low Ionic Strength (Salt) Solution*

PRP = *Platelet Rich Plasma*

SOPs = *Standard Operating Procedures*

Appendix 3:
Recommendations/Resolutions of the Council of Europe in the field of blood transfusion

Resolution (78) 29
> on the harmonisation of legislations of member States relating to removal, grafting and transplantation of human substances

Recommendation No. R (79) 5
> on the transport and international exchange of substances of human origin

Recommendation No. R (80) 5
> on blood products for the treatment of haemophiliacs

Recommendation No. R (81) 5
> on antenatal administration of anti-D immunoglobulin

Recommendation No. R (81) 14
> on the assessment of the risks of transmitting infectious diseases by international transfer of blood, its components and derivatives

Recommendation No. R (83) 8
> on preventing the possible transmission of acquired immune deficiency syndrome (AIDS) from affected blood to patients receiving blood or blood products

Recommendation No. R (84) 6
> on prevention of the transmission of malaria by blood transfusion

Recommendation No. R (85) 5
> on the study on the current position of training programmes for future specialists in blood transfusion in Council of Europe member states and in Finland

Recommendation No. R (85) 12
> on the screening of blood donors for the presence of Aids markers

Recommendation No. R (86) 6
> on the guidelines for the preparation, quality control and use of fresh frozen plasma (FFP)

Recommendation No. R (87) 25
> on the common European public health policy to fight the acquired immunodeficiency syndrome (AIDS)

Recommendation No. R (88) 4
> on the responsibilities of health authorities in the field of blood transfusion

Recommendation No. R (90) 3
> on medical research on human beings

Recommendation No. R (90) 9
> on plasma products and European self-sufficiency

Recommendation No. R (93) 4
> on clinical trials involving the use of components and fractionated products derived from human blood or plasma

Recommendation No. R (95) 14
> on the protection of the health of donors and recipients in the area of blood transfusion

Resolution 812 (1983)
> of the Parliamentary Assembly on Aids

Recommendation No. R (96) 11
> on documentation and record-keeping to guarantee the traceability of blood and blood products especially in hospital

Recommendation No. R (98) 2
> on provision of haematopoietic progenitor cells

Recommendation No. R (98) 10
> on the use of human red blood cells for preparation of oxygen carrying substances

Recommendation Rec(2001)4
> on the possible transmission of variant Creutzfeldt-Jakob Disease (vCJD) by blood transfusion

Recommendation Rec(2002)11
> on the hospital's and clinician's role in the optimal use of blood and blood products

Recommendation Rec(2003)11
> on the introduction of pathogen inactivation procedures for blood components

Recommendation Rec(2004)8
> on autologous cord blood banks

Recommendation Rec(2004)18
> on teaching transfusion medicine to nurses

N.B.　　The figures in brackets indicate the year of adoption by the Committee of Ministers

Appendix 4: List of publications

1976   Production and use of cellular blood components for transfusion
Study Director: B. Bucher with M. Benbunan, H. Heisto, U. Reesink

1978   Indications for the use of albumin, plasmaprotein solutions and plasma substitutes
Study Director: J. O'Riordan with M. Aebischer, J. Darnborough and I. Thoren

1980   Preparation and use of coagulation factors VIII and IX for transfusion
Study Director: R. Masure with G. Myllyla, I. Temperley and Stampli

1981   Assessment of the risks of transmitting infectious diseases by international transfer of blood, its components and derivatives
Study Director: W. Weise with T. Nielsen, P. Skinhot, J.P. Saleun

1982   European Co-operation in the field of blood: miscellany reports on the occasion of the 20th anniversary of the Committee of Experts on blood transfusion and Immunohaematology 1962-1982
P. Cazal, A. André, P. Lundsgaard-Hansen, W. Weise, R. Butler, C.P. Engelfriet, and A. Hässig

1983   Essential aspects of tissue typing
B. Bradley and S. Gore

1985   Study on the current position of training programmes for future specialists in blood transfusion in Council of Europe member states and in Finland
Study Director: E. Freiesleben with A. André, A. Franco, B. Baysal, J. Cash.

1986   Quality control in blood transfusion services
Study Director: E. Freiesleben, R. Butler, C. Hogman, W. Wagstaff

1987   Renal transplantation: sense and sensitisation
B. Bradley and S. Gore, Martinus Nijhoff Publishers

1988   First European Symposium on quality in blood transfusion
Résumé of lectures (publication of the Health Division of the Council of Europe)

1989   European Course on Blood transfusion (Athens, March 1988)
        Compendium of lecturers (publication of the Health Division of the
        Council of Europe)

1990   Blood transfusion: 2nd European Course (Madrid 1990)
        Compendium of lecturers (publication of the Health Division of the
        Council of Europe)

1992   Impact of the Aids epidemic on health care services and planning
        in Europe (publication of the Health Division of the Council of
        Europe)

1992   Plasma products and European self-sufficiency: collection,
        preparation and use
        Study Director: J. Leikola with W. van Aken, C. Hogman, D. Lee, M.
        Muglia, H. Schmitt

1993   Blood transfusion in Europe: a "white paper". Safe and sufficient
        blood in Europe by Piet J Hagen

1993   Survey of blood transfusion services of central and eastern
        European countries and their co-operation with western
        transfusion services
        Report by H.T. Heiniger

1993   The collection and use of human blood and plasma in Europe
        by Prof. Dr. W G Van Aken

1995   Guide on the Preparation, use and quality assurance in blood
        components (appendix to Recommendation No. R (95) 15)

1997   Collection and use of blood and plasma in Europe (member States
        of the Council of Europe not members of the European Union)
        Study 1995
        Report by Dr Rejman

1997   Activities of blood banks in relation to bone marrow
        transplantations
        Study Director: I.M. Francklin; Group members S. Koskimies, R.
        Kroczek,
        M. Reti, L. de Waal, R. Arrieta, F. Carbonell-Uberos

1998   Blood transfusion : half a century of contribution by the Council of
        Europe
        Report by Prof. Dr B. Genetet

2000   Collection and use of human blood and plasma in the non-European
        Union Council of Europe member States in 1997
        Report by Dr Rejman

2000   Autologous blood donation and transfusion in Europe – 1997 data
        Report by Prof. Politis

2001   Pathogen inactivation of labile blood products
        Study Director: Prof. A. Morell

2002   Autologous blood donation and transfusion in Europe – 2000 data
        Report by Prof. Politis

2004   Collection, testing and use of blood and blood products in Europe –
        2001 data
        Report by Dr van der Poel

2005   Collection, testing and use of blood and blood products in Europe –
        2002 data
        Report by Dr van der Poel

Index

A

B

H

I

L

M

P

Q

R

S

T

Z

Sales agents for publications of the Council of Europe
Agents de vente des publications du Conseil de l'Europe

BELGIUM/BELGIQUE
La Librairie européenne
Rue de l'Orme 1
B-1040 BRUXELLES
Tel.: (32) 2 231 04 35
Fax: (32) 2 735 08 60
E-mail: mail@libeurop.be
http://www.libeurop.be

Jean de Lannoy
202, avenue du Roi
B-1190 BRUXELLES
Tel.: (32) 2 538 4308
Fax: (32) 2 538 0841
E-mail: jean.de.lannoy@euronet.be
http://www.jean-de-lannoy.be

CANADA
Renouf Publishing Company Limited
5369 Chemin Canotek Road
CDN-OTTAWA, Ontario, K1J 9J3
Tel.: (1) 613 745 2665
Fax: (1) 613 745 7660
E-mail: order.dept@renoufbooks.com
http://www.renoufbooks.com

CZECH REP./RÉP. TCHÈQUE
Suweco Cz Dovoz Tisku Praha
Ceskomoravska 21
CZ-18021 PRAHA 9
Tel.: (420) 2 660 35 364
Fax: (420) 2 683 30 42
E-mail: import@suweco.cz

DENMARK/DANEMARK
GAD Direct
Fiolstæde 31-33
DK-1171 KOBENHAVN K
Tel.: (45) 33 13 72 33
Fax: (45) 33 12 54 94
E-mail: info@gaddirect.dk

FINLAND/FINLANDE
Akateeminen Kirjakauppa
Keskuskatu 1, PO Box 218
FIN-00381 HELSINKI
Tel.: (358) 9 121 41
Fax: (358) 9 121 4450
E-mail: akatilaus@stockmann.fi
http://www.akatilaus.akateeminen.com

GERMANY/ALLEMAGNE
AUSTRIA/AUTRICHE
UNO Verlag
August Bebel Allee 6
D-53175 BONN
Tel.: (49) 2 28 94 90 20
Fax: (49) 2 28 94 90 222
E-mail: bestellung@uno-verlag.de
http://www.uno-verlag.de

GREECE/GRÈCE
Librairie Kauffmann
Mavrokordatou 9
GR-ATHINAI 106 78
Tel.: (30) 1 38 29 283
Fax: (30) 1 38 33 967
E-mail: ord@otenet.gr

HUNGARY/HONGRIE
Euro Info Service
Hungexpo Europa Kozpont ter 1
H-1101 BUDAPEST
Tel.: (361) 264 8270
Fax: (361) 264 8271
E-mail: euroinfo@euroinfo.hu
http://www.euroinfo.hu

ITALY/ITALIE
Libreria Commissionaria Sansoni
Via Duca di Calabria 1/1, CP 552
I-50125 FIRENZE
Tel.: (39) 556 4831
Fax: (39) 556 41257
E-mail: licosa@licosa.com
http://www.licosa.com

NETHERLANDS/PAYS-BAS
De Lindeboom Internationale
Publicaties b.v.
M.A. de Ruyterstraat 20 A
NL-7482 BZ HAAKSBERGEN
Tel.: (31) 53 574 0004
Fax: (31) 53 572 9296
E-mail: books@delindeboom.com
http://www.delindeboom.com

NORWAY/NORVÈGE
Akademika A/S Universitetsbokhandel
PO Box 84, Blindern
N-0314 OSLO
Tel.: (47) 22 85 30 30
Fax: (47) 23 12 24 20

POLAND/POLOGNE
Głowna Księgarnia Naukowa
im. B. Prusa
Krakowskie Przedmiescie 7
PL-00-068 WARSZAWA
Tel.: (48) 29 22 66
Fax: (48) 22 26 64 49
E-mail: inter@internews.com.pl
http://www.internews.com.pl

PORTUGAL
Livraria Portugal
Rua do Carmo, 70
P-1200 LISBOA
Tel.: (351) 13 47 49 82
Fax: (351) 13 47 02 64
E-mail: liv.portugal@mail.telepac.pt

SPAIN/ESPAGNE
Mundi-Prensa Libros SA
Castelló 37
E-28001 MADRID
Tel.: (34) 914 36 37 00
Fax: (34) 915 75 39 98
E-mail: libreria@mundiprensa.es
http://www.mundiprensa.com

SWITZERLAND/SUISSE
Adeco – Van Diermen
Chemin du Lacuez 41
CH-1807 BLONAY
Tel.: (41) 21 943 26 73
Fax: (41) 21 943 36 05
E-mail: info@adeco.org

UNITED KINGDOM/
ROYAUME-UNI
TSO (formerly HMSO)
51 Nine Elms Lane
GB-LONDON SW8 5DR
Tel.: (44) 207 873 8372
Fax: (44) 207 873 8200
E-mail: customer.services@theso.co.uk
http://www.the-stationery-office.co.uk
http://www.itsofficial.net

UNITED STATES and CANADA/
ÉTATS-UNIS et CANADA
Manhattan Publishing Company
468 Albany Post Road, PO Box 850
CROTON-ON-HUDSON,
NY 10520, USA
Tel.: (1) 914 271 5194
Fax: (1) 914 271 5856
E-mail: Info@manhattanpublishing.com
http://www.manhattanpublishing.com

———————

FRANCE
La Documentation française
(Diffusion/Vente France entière)
124 rue H. Barbusse
93308 Aubervilliers Cedex
Tel.: (33) 01 40 15 70 00
Fax: (33) 01 40 15 68 00
E-mail: vel@ladocfrancaise.gouv.fr
http://www.ladocfrancaise.gouv.fr

Librairie Kléber (Vente Strasbourg)
Palais de l'Europe
F-67075 Strasbourg Cedex
Fax: (33) 03 88 52 91 21
E-mail: librairie.kleber@coe.int

Council of Europe Publishing/Editions du Conseil de l'Europe
F-67075 Strasbourg Cedex
Tel.: (33) 03 88 41 25 81 – Fax: (33) 03 88 41 39 10 – E-mail: publishing@coe.int – Website: http://book.coe.int